Hereditas Archaeologica Hungariae

2.

Series editors

Elek Benkő, Erzsébet Jerem, Gyöngyi Kovács, József Laszlovszky

Adrienn Papp

THE TURKISH BATHS OF HUNGARY: ARCHAEOLOGICAL REMAINS OF THE OTTOMAN ERA

ARCHAEOLINGUA

MTA
Bölcsészettudományi
Kutatóközpont
Régészeti Intézet

Budapest 2018

The publication of this volume was funded by generous grants from the National Cultural Fund of Hungary, the Book and Journal Publishing Committee of the Hungarian Academy of Sciences, the Research Centre for the Humanities of the Hungarian Academy of Sciences, and the Budapest History Museum

Nemzeti Kulturális Alap

MTA Bölcsészettudományi Kutatóközpont

BUDAPESTI TÖRTÉNETI MÚZEUM BTM

Cover photo:
The Ottoman era hot room of the Rudas Baths in Buda today

Volume editor: Gyöngyi Kovács

English translation: Michael James Webb
Copy editor: Zsuzsanna Renner
Editorial assistant: Ágnes Drosztmér
Desktop editing and layout: Zsuzsanna Kiss
Series and cover design: Móni Kaszta

ISBN 978-615 5766 05 3
HU ISSN 2498-5600

2018

ARCHAEOLINGUA FOUNDATION
H-1067 Budapest, Teréz krt. 13.
www.archaeolingua.hu
Managing Director: Erzsébet Jerem

Printed in Hungary by AduPrint Nyomda és Kiadó Kft.

Table of Contents

Editors' Foreword

The Turkish baths in Hungary occupy a special place in Hungary's archaeological heritage. These are buildings that we are still using for the function they were originally designed, and–especially in today's Budapest–they are viewed as part of modern bathing culture. At the same time, these buildings are not mere venues for physical rest and recreation, they are historical documents of an era, relics of the period and its culture. The Ottoman occupation in Hungary was in many respects a sad and destructive period in Hungarian history. However, there are a number of phenomena, even in modern everyday life, that can be traced back to external influences on our Hungarian homeland. One need only think of bathing or coffee.

The medieval Hungarian thermal water baths were replaced by a great many more Turkish baths during the Occupation era, and where there were no hot water springs the bath-houses were equipped with heating. We are able to envisage these from the preserved remains of our built heritage. In many cases, archaeology has exposed these relics or has demonstrated that within modern structures parts of Ottoman buildings lay hidden. The results of Hungarian heritage conservation and archaeological research are also important in the international context, many remains have been preserved, excavated or at least documented. One particularly important advance has been the archaeological research and analysis into monuments linked to written sources. Of course, this applies not only to baths but also to other typical buildings of the period under review, including mosques, minarets and mausoleums.

The surge of archaeological investigations into Ottoman buildings that took place in Hungary several decades ago gave fresh momentum to the archaeological excavations carried out during renovations on several important bath buildings over the past decade. This has also provided an opportunity to summarize the knowledge that has been accumulating since the end of the 17th century: data from the first surveys of buildings, from architects and researchers in the field of conservation and survey of monuments, and the generations of historians struggling with the not insignificant difficulties of written sources and archaeological excavation specialists. Consequently, it was this topic we chose when designing the second volume of the Hungarian archaeological heritage series. These monuments show superbly how a building can be both a part of architectural heritage and of modern everyday life. The presentation of the baths, however, is not just a description of the main historical data, architectural features and phenomena discovered during the excavations, but also points to the connections and contexts that illustrate many characteristic features of this historical period.

Elek Benkő, Erzsébet Jerem, Gyöngyi Kovács, József Laszlovszky

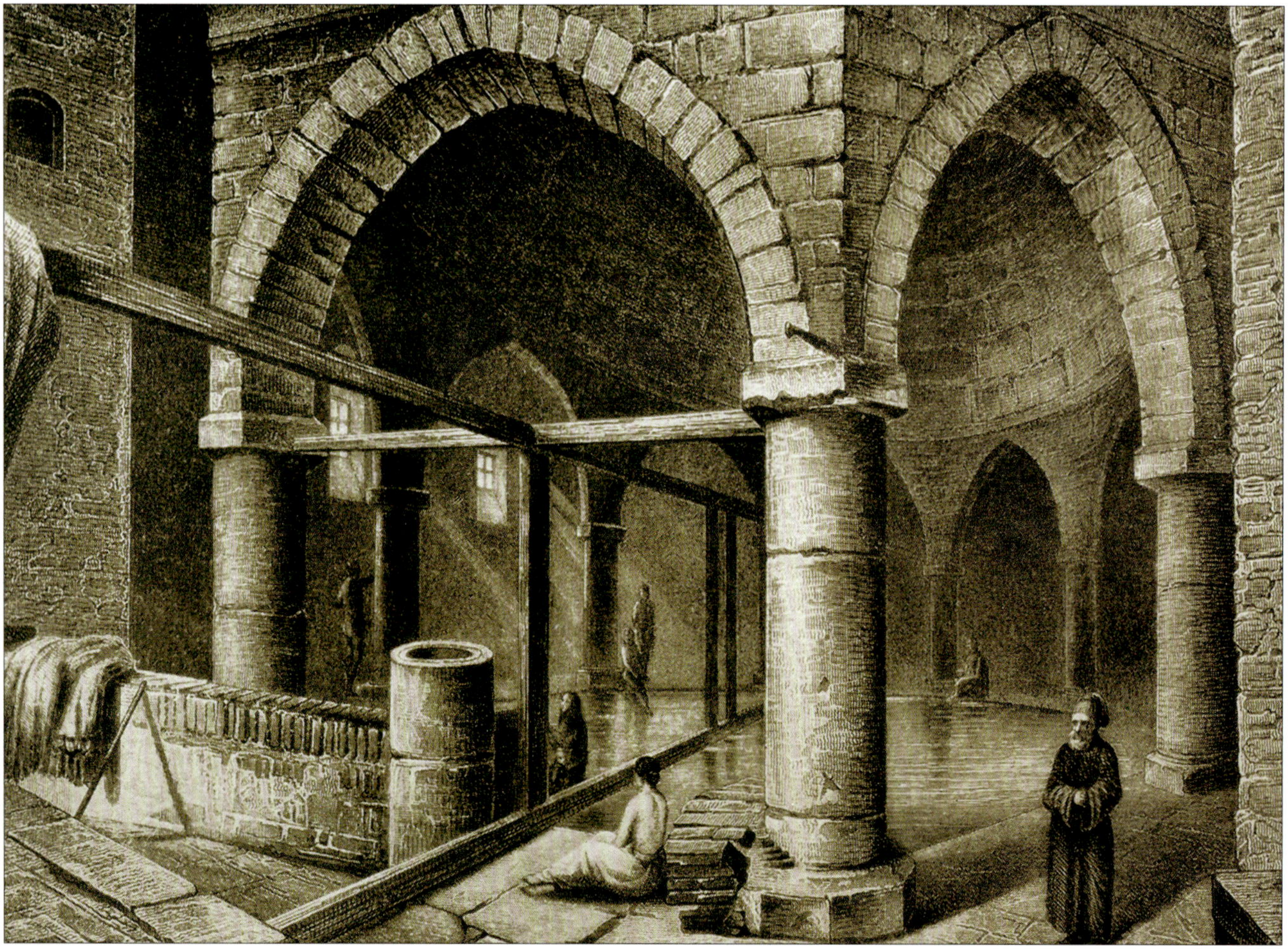

Figure 1. The hot room of the Rudas Baths in Buda in an engraving by Ludwig Rohbock, 1859

Introduction

Hungary has always been famous for its thermal springs, most of the travellers arriving today visit one or other of the country's baths. In centuries past, this was also the case. In the era of the Ottoman occupation, many travel stories praised the beneficial effects of the Hungarian baths. We hear of frostbitten travellers warming their fingers and toes, and also of local women seeking a cure. In my book, bath culture is introduced through this period (1541–1699), embedded within the context of Ottoman architecture. In the territories conquered by the Turks, thermal baths were built over natural hot springs. Among these are the buildings that have been used since that time, i.e. for almost 450 years (*Figure 1*). At the same time, steam baths were established across the region, but these have been destroyed and can only be explored with archaeological methods. The system of steam baths and bathing habits in these baths (*hamams*) seem very unusual to us because they have never had pools. Yet they were among the most characteristic and most widespread buildings of the era. In this volume I describe the general characteristics of Turkish baths and how they are used. Anyone who would like to try out how these baths worked centuries ago can do so by visiting today's Turkey because in Turkish areas the use of the spa remains unchanged.

In addition to this, the reader can acquaint themselves with the ancient monuments of Hungary: those buildings or ruins that have been explored through modern research. The bath buildings of the 16th-17th centuries are a perfect example. On the one hand, the design of the domed rooms themselves required a great deal of knowledge. On the other hand, the piping of water to the proper places, and the development of the underfloor heating system in the steam baths all demonstrate significant knowledge. Some of Buda's buildings rival the Sultan and Grand Vizier baths of Istanbul in their size and beauty. They were built in the heyday of the Ottoman Empire and represent its classical architectural style. The columns supporting the dome at the Rudas Bath in Buda and the emblematic chambers of the Császár Baths are the outstanding creations of the era. I could lead the Buda research personally, so it is those baths I have the most detailed knowledge of. Among them, we find the best-preserved Turkish baths, which are important architectural monuments in today's Budapest, and outstanding assets in terms of tourism.

In this volume you can learn about the remains of a period, many of the written sources for which were recorded with Arabic letters. For this, the international scientific community uses a unique system for transcription. However, the Turkish names and phrases that appear in this volume are, for the sake of easier readability, written according to the English spelling rules as they generally are in international research work.

In the Hungarian language "Turkish occupation" and "the conquering Turks" have become specific terms by which the 16th-century Ottoman expansion is understood. This is evidence of the significant historical impact that Ottoman conquest had on the Hungarian people. The Turks are in fact more than one nation, speaking several languages, of which one is today's Turkey and the Anatolian Turks. In Central Asia many other Turkish peoples live in a history in which there are other great empires similar to the Ottoman Empire.

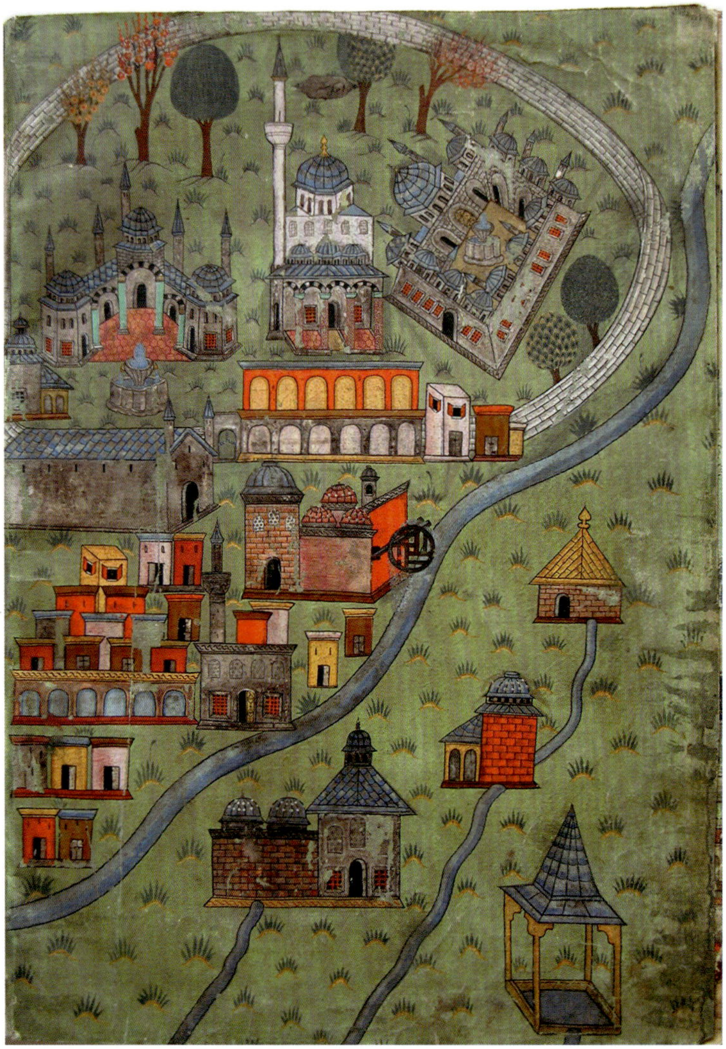

Figure 2. An Anatolian town (Eskişehir). Representation by Matrakchi Nasuh with characteristic Ottoman buildings, 16th century. Baths can be seen in the foreground and the centre of the picture.

I. The Ottoman Empire

The central part of the mediaeval Kingdom of Hungary was occupied by a major eastern power, the Ottoman Empire, for almost one hundred and fifty years.

In the 16th century, at the height of its powers, the Ottoman Empire was one of the period's most significant political factors. Its eastern borders were in the western region of present-day Iran, and it also governed the North African shore of the Mediterranean all the way to Algeria. A mere fifty years previously, it had been a much smaller state extending no further than Anatolya to the east; while to the west, its borders lay at the Adriatic, and to the North its territory extended into the Kingdom of Hungary (*Figures 2-3*).

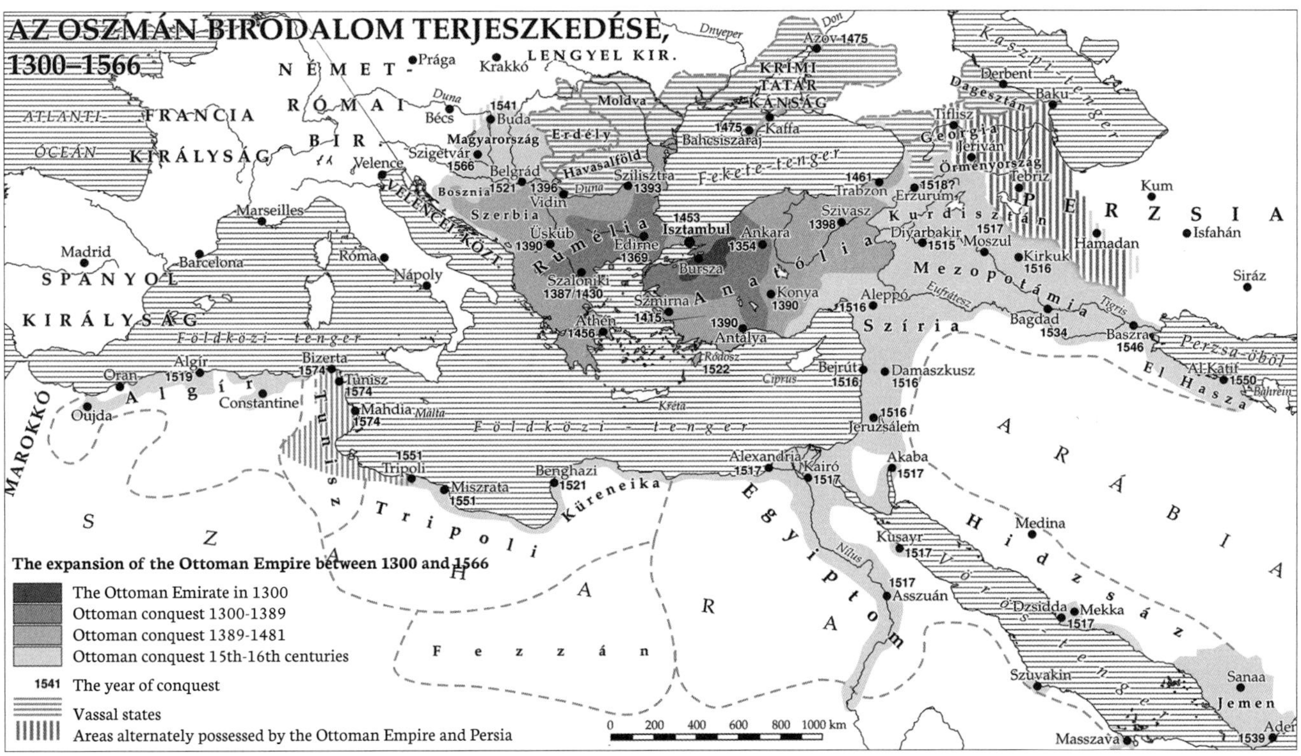

Figure 3. The expansion of the Ottoman Empire until 1566

The foundations of this explosively developing and growing empire were laid by Turkic tribes migrating from Central Asia towards the west that began to enter the territory of the Byzantine Empire in the 11th century. Their first large state, which reached from the Aegean Sea to Central Asia, was established under the Seljuk dynasty in the 11th century. By the 13th century, this empire had disintegrated beneath the barrage of blows dealt it by the Mongols, and smaller emirates (*beylik* in Turkish) were established in Anatolya. One of them was a small state ruled by Osman, established near the Sea of Marmara close to the Byzantine border. The eponymous founder of the new dynasty, Osman I (died 1323/24), ruled over just a small area, but under the reign of his son, Orhan, the beylik grew to be a significant power within Anatolya. They occupied important Byzantine territories, including the southern shores of the Sea of Marmara and, in particular, in 1326, the city of Bursa, which became the sultanate's capital for a brief period. In the middle of the 14th century, it also gained a foothold on the European continent, while their conquests proceeded in parallel both in the Balkans and in Anatolya. The constantly growing state retained Constantinople and its surroundings as a relic of the diminishing Byzantine Empire embedded within it.

The almost constant expansion came to a halt in 1402 when the Ottomans found themselves face to face with Tamerlane, the most important Central Asian conqueror of the period. The heartland of Tamerlane's empire, which at the time extended from India to Anatolya, was in the Amu Darya - Syr Darya region. The Ottoman Sultanate's sovereign, Bayezid I, battled Tamerlane's armies in 1402 at Ankara, suffering a decisive defeat. The sultan was captured and remained a prisoner for the rest of his days. Tamerlane ransacked Anatolya and re-established the small emirates. The Ottoman expansion was halted for almost half a century, only to continue then with renewed vigour. Mehmed II conquered Constantinople in 1453 and established the new capital of his empire there. Through further conquests in the 16th century, the Middle East, North Africa and Arabia, considered to be the sacred heart of the Islamic world, were all added to the Ottoman Empire. A few decades later, the middle section of the Kingdom of Hungary was also occupied. Although that territory was lost by the end of the 17th century, the Ottoman Empire retained most of its massive range until the middle of the 19th century. It only came to lose the decisive majority of its territories in the Balkans and in Africa in the late 19th and early 20th centuries. The last Ottoman Sultan, Mehmed IV, went into exile in 1922.

II. Ottoman Hungary

The explosive growth of the Ottoman Empire coincided with its attacks upon the Kingdom of Hungary. While the sultans could boast of massive conquests in the Middle East and in Africa, in the West its expansion was halted at the Kingdom of Hungary, and the sultanate would never occupy the kingdom as a whole. Conflicts between the two states had begun in the 14th century. At the Battle of Nicopolis in 1396, the army of King Sigismund of Luxemburg was routed. As a result, the Hungarian political elite recognised the importance of the southern line of defence and the significance of its southern neighbours—Bosnia, Serbia and Wallachia—in the war against the Ottoman Empire.

The southern system of border fortifications passed with flying colours at the 1456 Battle of Belgrade. During the reign of Sultan Süleyman (1520-1566), the front line shifted into the territory of the Hungarian Kingdom. In 1521, Belgrade was lost, and in 1526, the Christian armies suffered a defeat at Mohács, deep within the country. The occupation of the middle section of the kingdom and the integration of that territory into the empire began several decades later, however, following the death of King John Zápolya and the fall of Buda (1541). From 1541 until the Treaty of Karlowitz, concluded in 1699, the struggle against the Ottoman Empire determined the life of the kingdom (*Figure 4*).

The parts of the Hungarian Kingdom that were carved off remained border country throughout, and the Hungarian Kingdom also continued to exist, albeit in a severely mutilated form. All of which resulted in a peculiar situation: the conquerors lived in fortified strongholds, while the population of the market-towns and villages between those points remained as it had been earlier, largely Hungarian. In the fortified towns, the number of locals gradually dwindled, and in many of those towns, none remained at all.

But who really were the conquerors that we are in the habit of calling Ottomans? The Southern Slavs fell on their feet under Ottoman rule, moving into the territories of the Hungarian Kingdom. Their fortunes are documented by surviving payroll accounts, for instance, and such data is confirmed by the Ottoman traveller of the era, Evliya Chelebi,[1] who recorded that most of the inhabitants spoke Bosnian to each other.[2] The majority of those moving to the occupied territories were soldiers, but a civilian population must also be taken into account: those people held some office in the religious institutions of Islam or in government administration, while another segment were artisans or traders. Local conditions were characterised by soldiers often engaging in civilian tasks as well as military. The conquerors did not call themselves Turks—at that time, such a thing would have been an insult—they much preferred the term 'Ottoman', thereby expressing their affiliation to the ruling dynasty and thus the empire. The culture of the elite was modelled on the Sultan's court, and used a language called 'Osmanli', essentially Turkish with many Persian and Arabic words and syntactic forms.

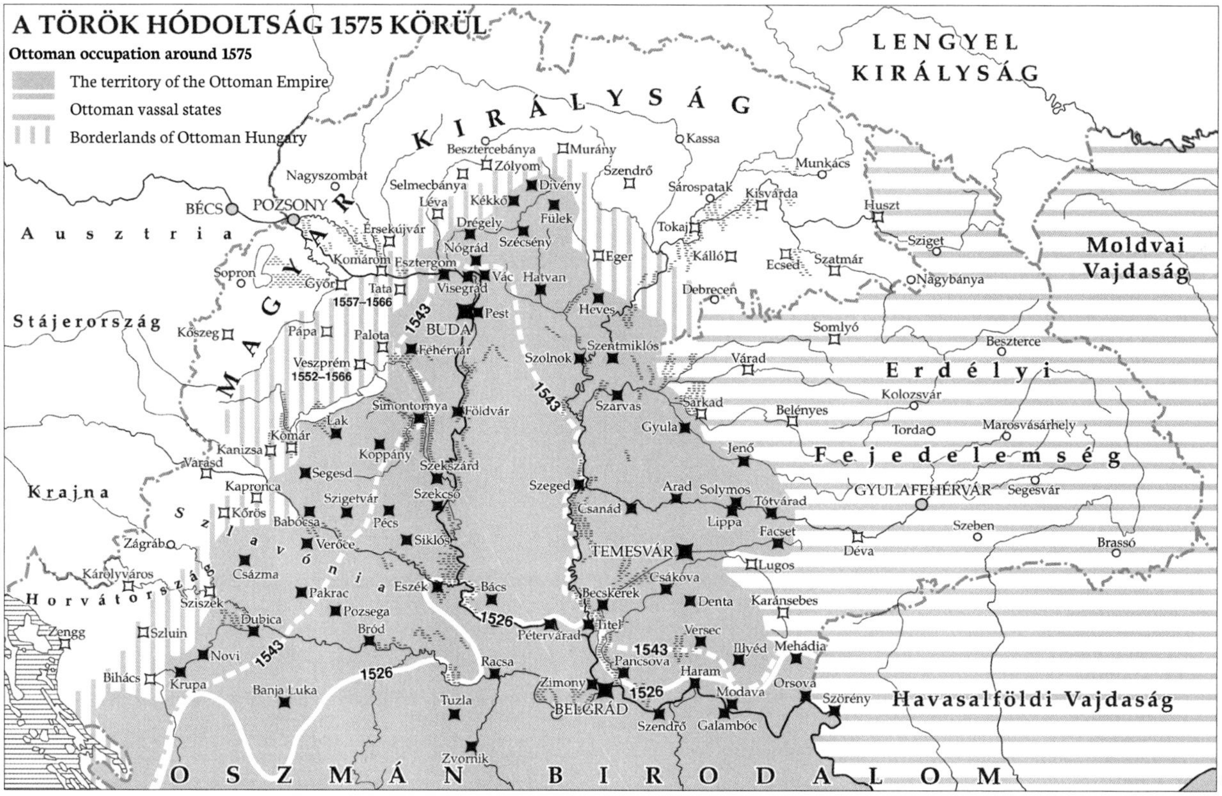

Figure 4. The Ottoman occupation around 1575

Ottoman society was fundamentally articulated into two strata. The first (the *askheri*) were the soldier class consisting of armed fighters, in addition to those performing legal, administrative and religious tasks; that is to say, everyone who received a salary from the state. The other class consisted of tax-paying artisans, traders and peasants, irrespective of their religious affiliation. A significant part of the elite—strange as that may sound to us—consisted of slaves who were delivered to a palace education through the system of *devshirme*, the 'tax payable in children'. The best among these were raised in the Sultan's *saray*, then entered a military or administrative profession to form the pillars of a government organisation loyal to the Sultan. In the course of their advancement, they were able to reach the highest position, that of grand vizier, indeed, in the classical age of the empire, the grand vizier's position could only be filled by a slave. The system was geared to producing a class of public servants who were loyal to the Sultan in all circumstances. Initially, the children to be enslaved were selected only from among the children of non-Muslims.

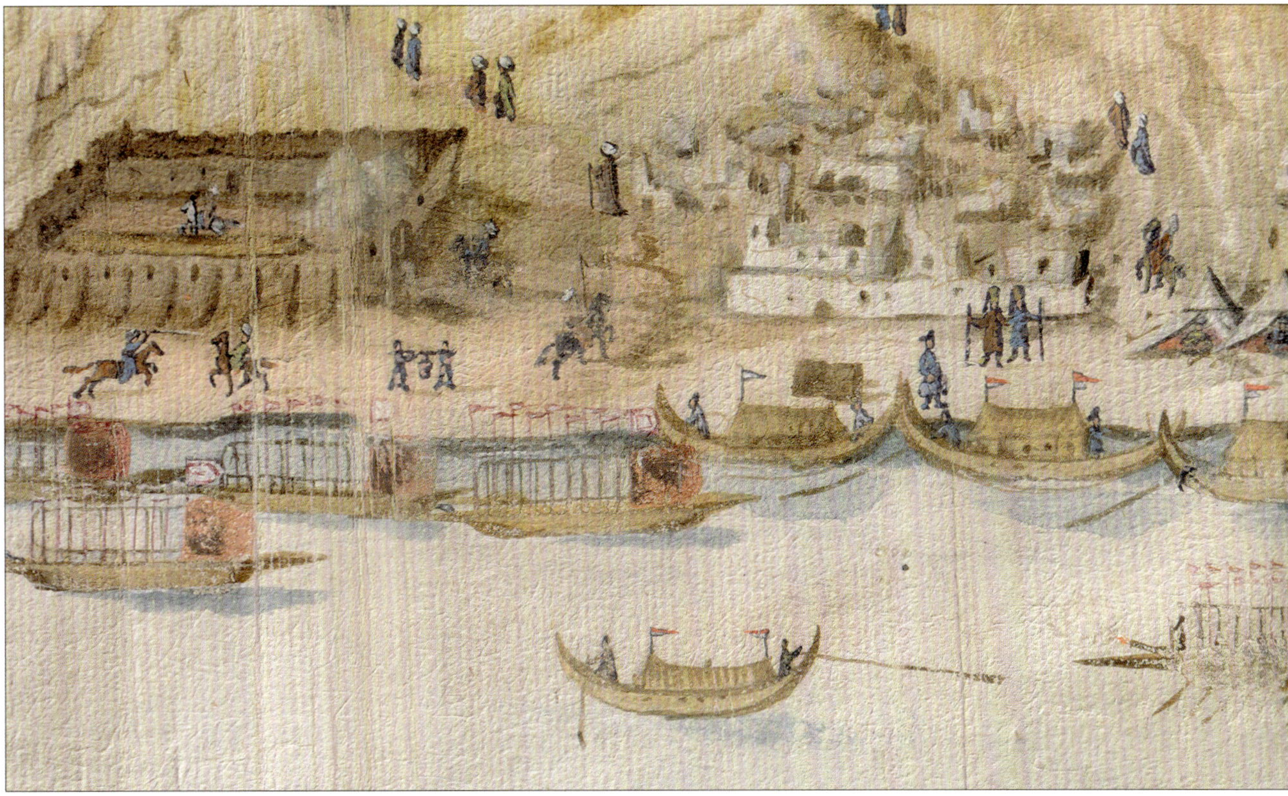

Figure 5. Ottoman soldiers. Section from a representation of Buda in watercolours, circa 1600

As the conquest progressed, the territories won over from the Hungarian Kingdom were organised into a number of districts (*vilayets*, with seats at Buda, Timișoara, Eger, Kanizsa, Várad and Nové Zámky), but the governor of the Buda *vilayet*, the Beylerbey of Buda, retained his paramount role throughout. The vilayets were divided into smaller administrative units known as *sanjaks*, and those in turn were divided into *nahiyes*. The populations of towns and villages were recorded to facilitate the levying of taxes and calculating anticipated incomes, before the beneficiary holdings were distributed and those remaining under the Sultan's direct management were also designated.

We now have only fragmentary information concerning the conquerors who arrived in the territory of the Kingdom of Hungary; and significantly more detailed knowledge exists about the soldiers stationed here (*Figure 5*)[3] than about the civilian population. Even so, it remains clear that the Ottomans spent sufficient time here for some families to put down roots, and to feel that the country was their home.[4]

The one hundred and fifty years of Ottoman rule constitute a period of Hungarian history rife with tribulations and with severe and extended consequences that coincided with its heyday and the early period of decline within the 600-year history of the Ottoman Empire. As in the Hungarian provinces, the period of Ottoman rule was clearly distinct from the Christian cultures of the previous and the succeeding periods from the perspective of the archaeological and architectural historical material of the country, it is also quite clear which items belong to the Ottoman period (*Figure 6*). Those artefacts present the classical Ottoman age with little or no outside influence.

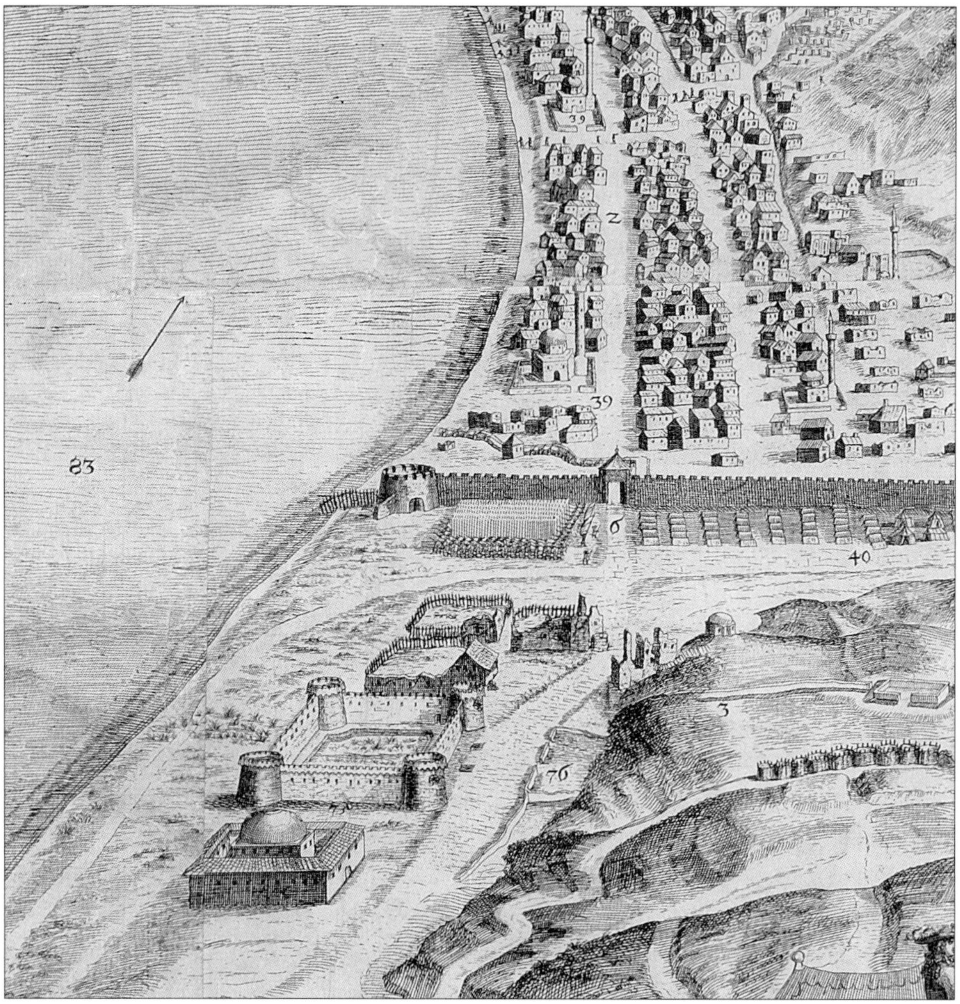

Figure 6. The area of the city around the Császár Baths at the end of the 17th century, including the fortress-like gunpowder mill and the mausoleum of Gül Baba on the hill. Below it, are the ruins of a monastery (*tekke*). An engraving of the 1686 siege of Buda by Domenico Fontana (detail)

III. The Heyday of Ottoman Architecture

The art of the Ottoman Empire was connected to the Sultan's palace by a number of threads (*Figure* 7). The artisanal workshops of the court played a definitive role in shaping it, and the styles created there spread throughout the empire. At times, the effect was direct: we know, for instance, that the faience workshops of Iznik received patterns from the Sultan's palace for the local artisans to paint onto objects that were ordered (*Figure 8*).

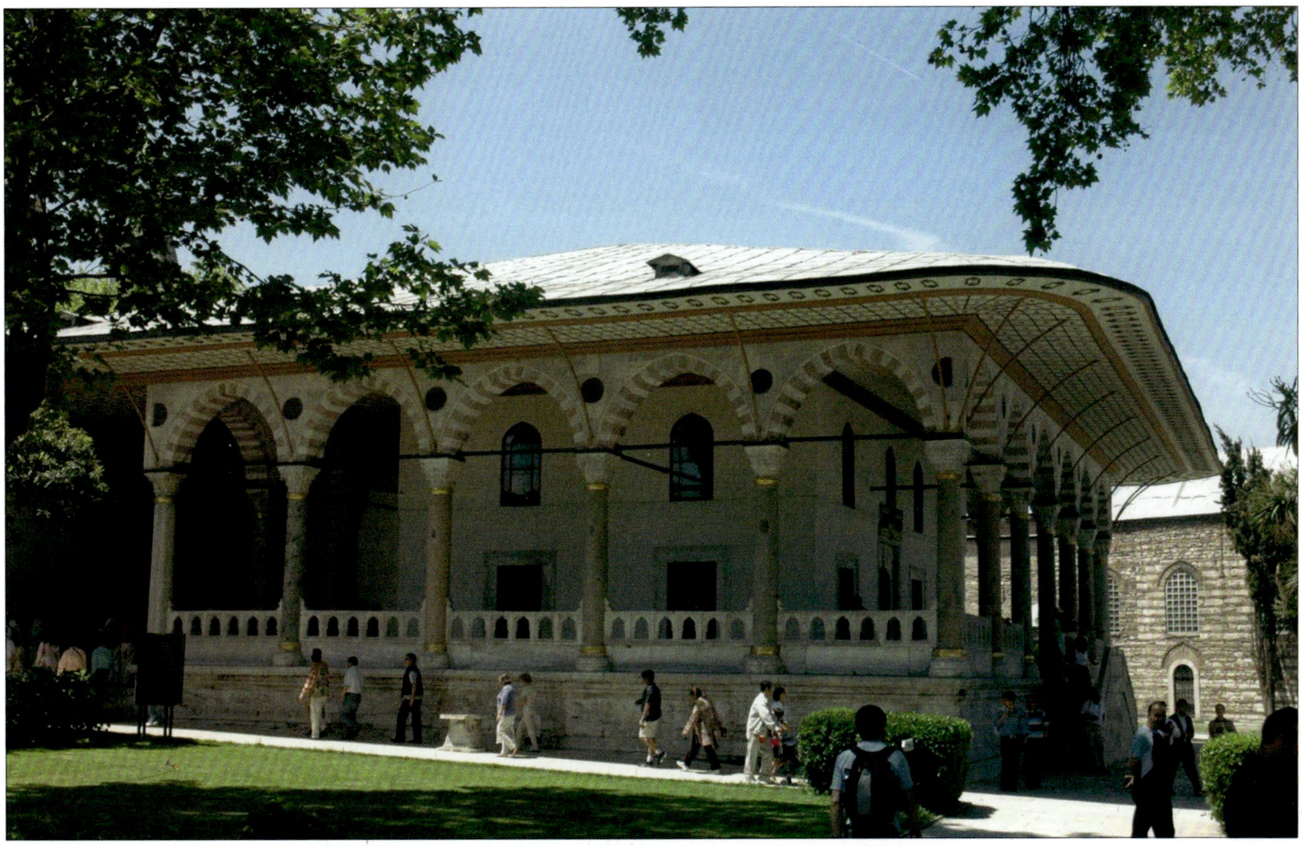

Figure 7. The Topkapi Palace Audience Chamber, Istanbul, 16th century

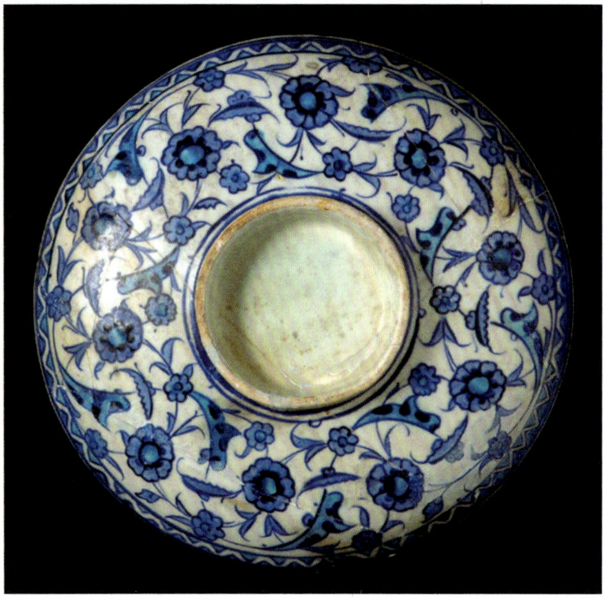

Figure 8. Iznik bowl from the golden age of Ottoman architecture, 16th century

Many of the court workshops were also connected with the Sultan's building projects. Under the leadership of the chief architect, the architects and the artisans under their command (carpenters, stonecutters, glassmakers, painters, etc.) formed a separate group. They were also trained in the court workshops, where those preparing for a career in architectural work would also study geometry, for example. During that period, architecture not only permitted the Ottoman elite to perform charitable deeds as prescribed by Islam (e.g. the foundation of mosques), but also to assert their position of power. Consequently, the kinds of building and where they were located were extremely important. One result of that was that mosques and schools (madrasas) were popping up all over Istanbul, while in the remoter corners of the empire where they were much needed they were in short supply. At the same time, due to strong centralisation and the tight links between the local Ottoman elite and Constantinople, even the remote provinces of the empire would follow Istanbul fashions, art forms and architectural patterns.

The greatest architect of the period, Mimar Sinan (*mimar* means 'architect'), was born into a Christian family in Kayseri, Central Turkey. He was sent to the court of the Sultan as 'child tax', although he was much older than was customary at almost twenty years old (he was born around 1490). Like all slave children, he was converted to Islam. He then studied to become a carpenter. Once his studies were completed he became a Janissary and travelled the length and breadth of the empire, encountering a wide range of military-architectural tasks. At Lake Van, for instance, he had to build a boat to cross the lake to obtain information about the hostile Safavid (Persian) army that was camped on the opposite shore.[5] In Moldova, he built a bridge over the Prut River for the Ottoman army. In 1538, in recognition of his knowledge, he was appointed chief architect to the empire. He remained in that position until his death at the age of one hundred in 1588. His biographies list some five hundred buildings as his work, which clearly indicates that a well-organised 'architectural office' must have been in operation. His projects determined the visual landscape of Ottoman Empire cities for a considerable period of time.

During that period, most Ottoman public buildings were dominated by domes, built in a variety of sizes, groups and configurations. The layout of buildings—their floor plans and their ornamentation—followed strict conventions. Before we begin to look at the baths, a review of the main types of building seems apposite.

The mosque

The patterns of Ottoman architecture were influenced very strongly by the Byzantine art of Constantinople. Anyone who stands between the Hagia Sophia (*Ayasofya*) and the Blue Mosque in Istanbul can have no doubt that the primary objective of Ottoman architecture was to outdo the 6th-century Byzantine Hagia Sophia. The grandiose mosques of the city are all highly varied expressions of that endeavour.

The individual types of building refer back to various earlier architectural traditions of the Islamic world, each with their own, specific characteristics.[6] The immediate precursors to the classical Ottoman era mosques were Christian churches built in the Byzantine Empire. The central square of their rectangular floor plans were covered by a dome. A number of the Sultan's mosques were built with huge domes and semidomes attached in order to span as large an area as possible. This block would have an adjacent enclosed yard, which was also usually square in outline, with a row of arcades lining its walls, covered in smaller domes in the case of particularly ornate buildings. In the centre of the yard there would be a well, the scene for ritual bathing. At a corner (or all corners) of the building, there are minarets, whose pencil shape also became a standard in Ottoman architecture from the 16th century.

In the case of smaller mosques simpler solutions are encountered: instead of a complex system of domes, the place of prayer may be spanned by a single dome or even a flat roof with small antechambers in front. Minarets were also built alongside such smaller buildings (*Figures 9-10*).

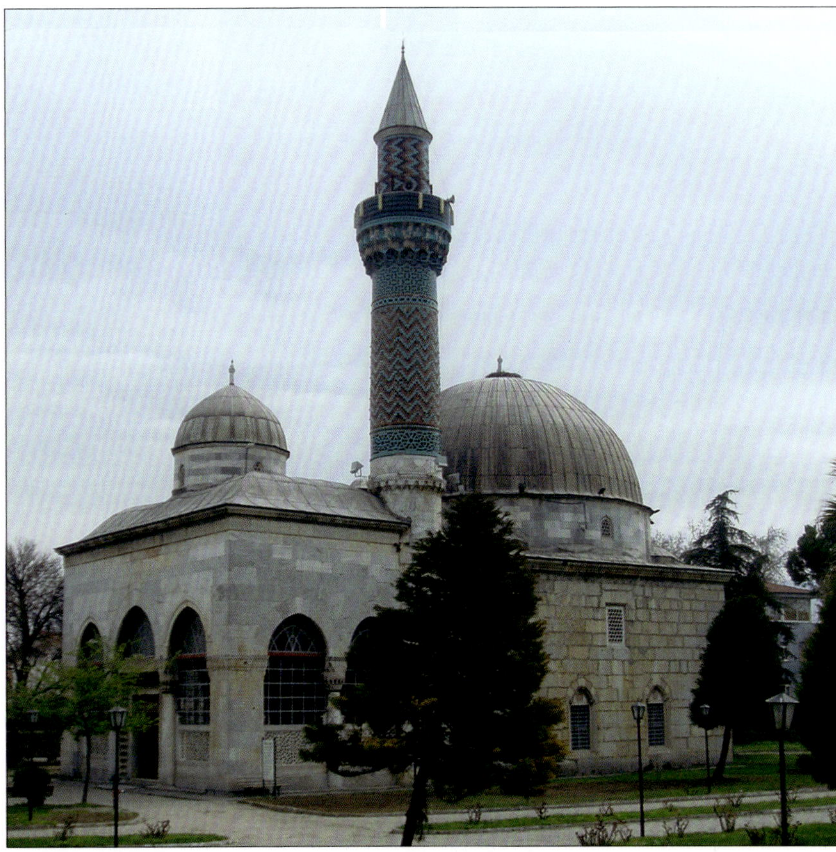

Figure 9. Smaller mosque with entrance hall, domes and minaret. Yeshil Mosque, Iznik, 1378-1391

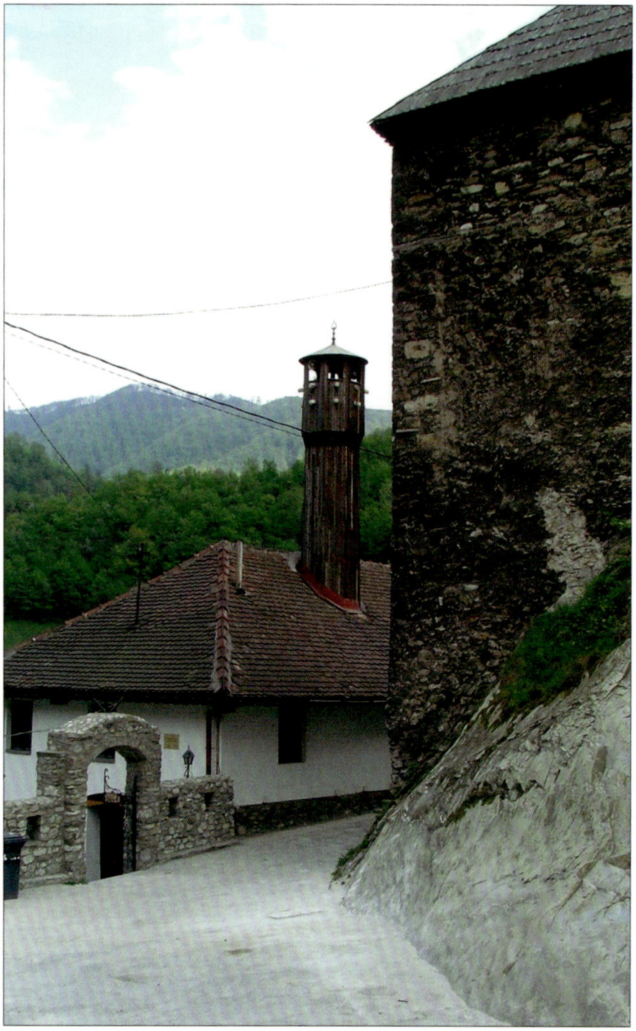

Figure 10. Simple hip-roofed mosque with wooden minaret. Vranduk, Bosnia, 15th century

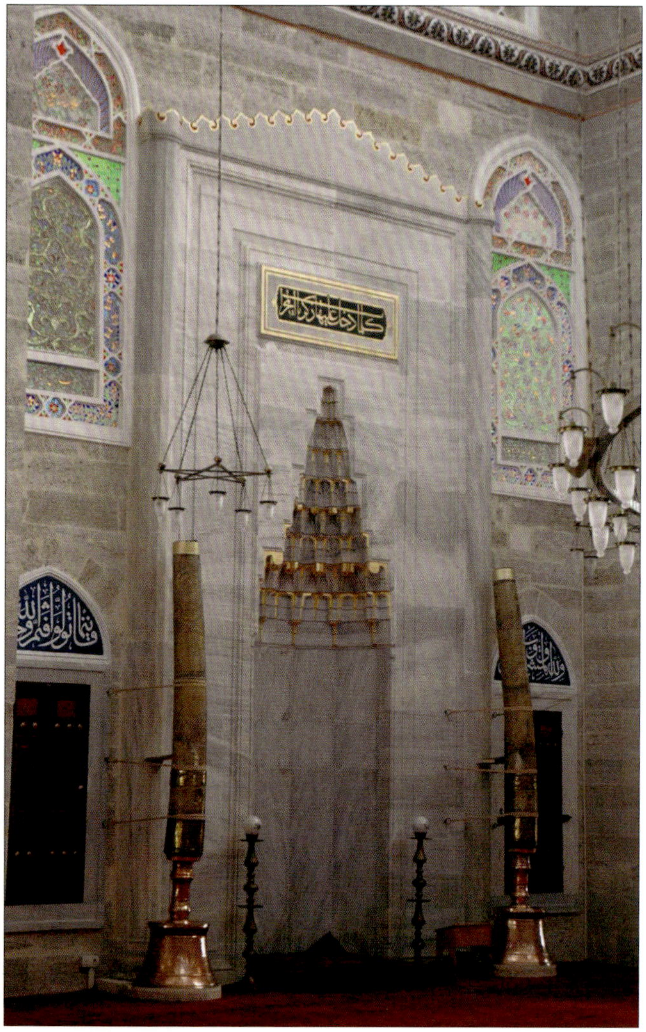

Figure 11. Mihrab in the Sultan Mihrimah Mosque, Istanbul, 1562-1565

Mosques also have some prerequisite elements of interior design which include the ornate niche in the wall that faces Mecca, the *mihrab* (*Figure 11*), intended to show the congregation the direction of Mecca, that is, the direction of their prayers. The pulpit (*minbar*) located next to the mihrab, used during Friday prayers, was usually made of wood or, occasionally, stone. Sultans and founders would often have special galleries built for them inside a mosque. The floors of mosques had carpets upon which the faithful would recite their prayers (*Figures 12-13*).

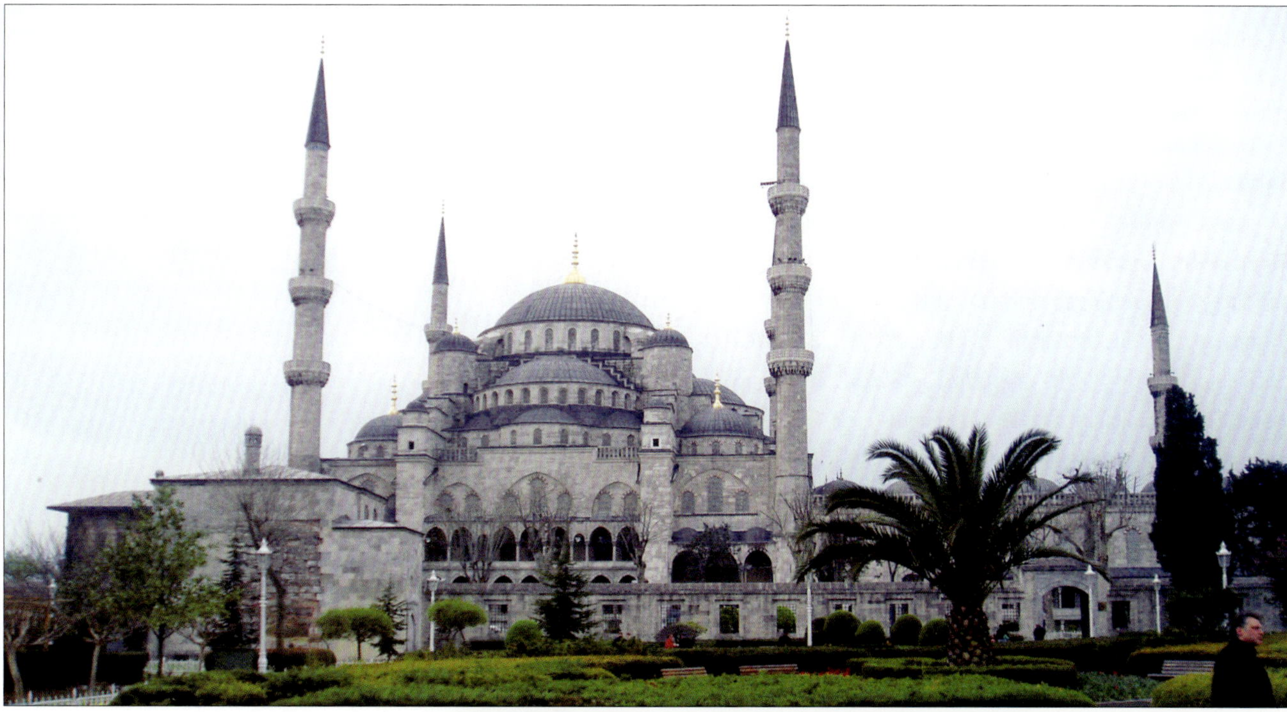

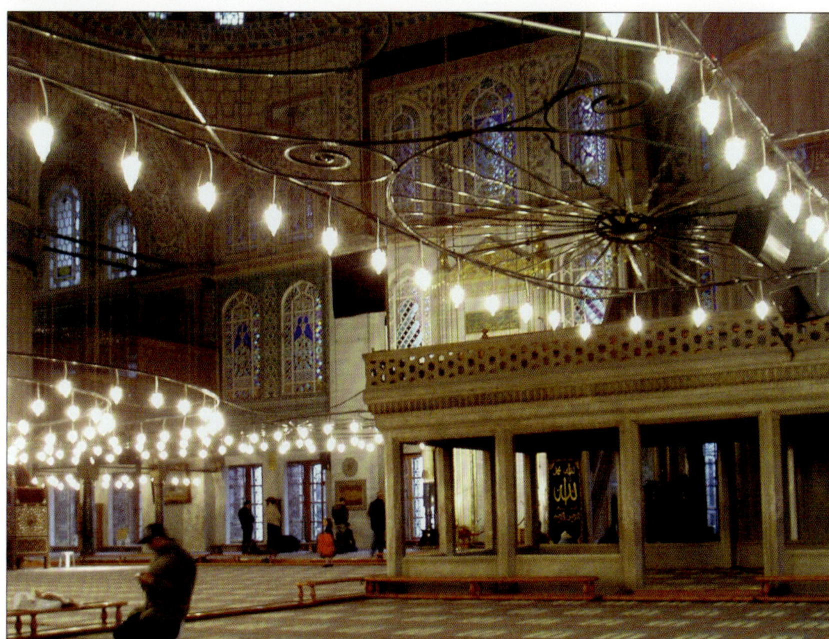

Figures 12-13. The Blue Mosque (Sultan Ahmed Mosque) in Istanbul and an interior view, 1609-1616

The madrasa

Madrasas were higher-level educational institutions for the study of Islam, at which—in contrast with Western European Universities—both the topics available and the depth to which they were studied were essentially determined by the teachers. Study of the Quran and religious law were the most important subjects, but medicine and natural sciences were also often included in the curriculum. A characteristic building type for madrasas developed in the Islamic world. During the classical age of Ottoman architecture, they were characterised by small rooms topped by domes arranged in a sequence surrounding a central yard. Generally, there would be an open corridor with columns in front of the rooms. The 'lecture hall' was located on the side opposite the entrance gate opening into the yard, although teaching could also occur in the yard itself, which would be ornamented with a fountain and plants (*Figure 14*).

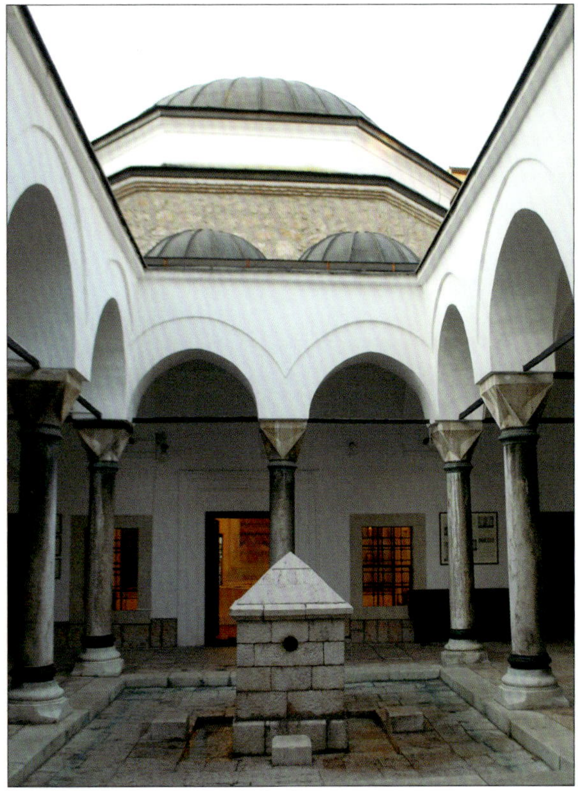

Figure 14. Inner courtyard of a madrasa (school). Kurshumliya Madrasa, Sarajevo, 1537

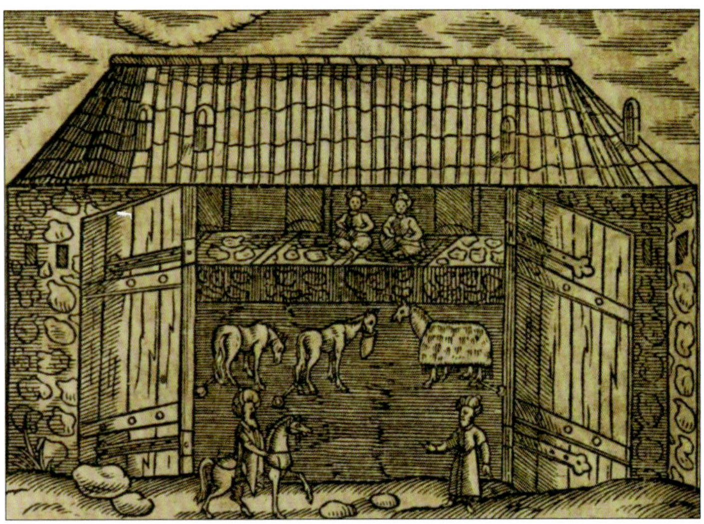

The caravanserai (*han*)

These multifunctional buildings essentially offered shelter and accommodation to traders and travellers within cities, and provided a venue for trading. They were usually rectangular, multi-storey buildings arranged around a courtyard. The traders lodged and offered their wares on the upper levels, while the ground floor was used for stabling animals (*Figure 15*).

Figure 15. Depiction of a caravanserai (inn) from the travel journal of Salomon Schweigger, 1639

The monastery (*tekke*)

The communities of Muslim monks (the dervishes) were not subject to the strict rules concerning the layout of structures that characterised other Ottoman building types or indeed Western European monasteries. Yet those buildings also exhibit a certain regularity, although they resemble residential buildings most closely. The buildings of a dervish monastery would be organised around several yards that were separated by walls. Gardens and the environment played an important role (*Figure 16*).

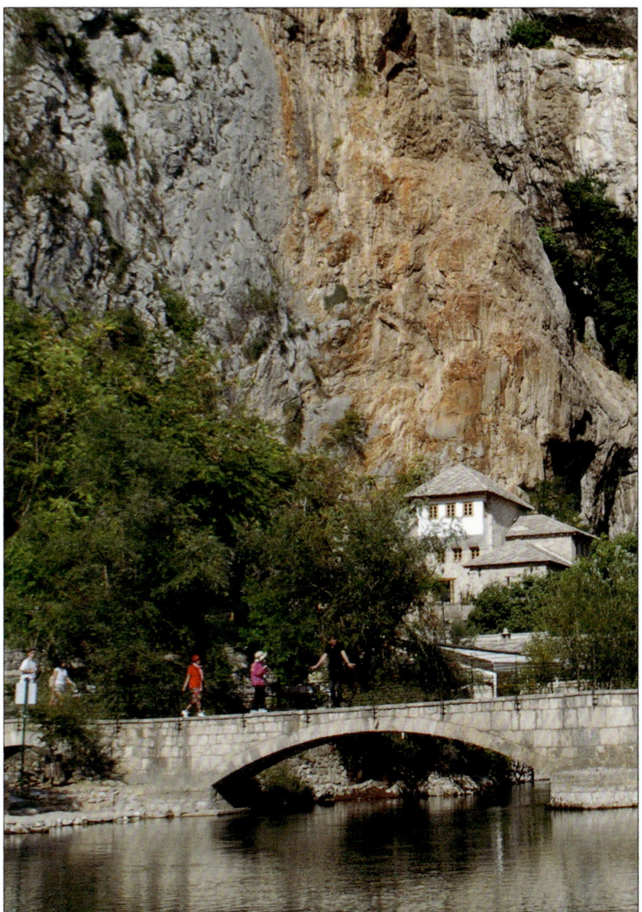

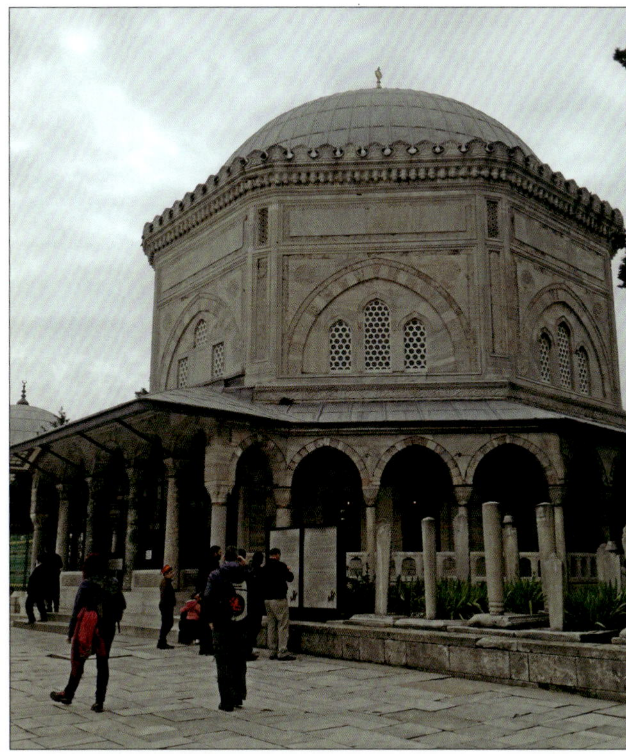

Figure 17. The mausoleum of Sultan Süleyman in Istanbul, 1550-1557

The mausoleum (*türbe*)

In Islamic architecture, mausoleums are stand-alone buildings with many common features but also some unique solutions in each region. Ottoman mausoleums are most commonly small and octagonal in layout, and covered by a dome. In some cases, a small projecting roof made of wood was installed over the entrance. The interior decoration of the Sultan's *türbes* (*Figure 17*) would often be lined with beautiful Iznik faience tiles.

Figure 16. Dervish monastery (*tekke*) in Blagaj, Bosnia, late 15th - early 16th century

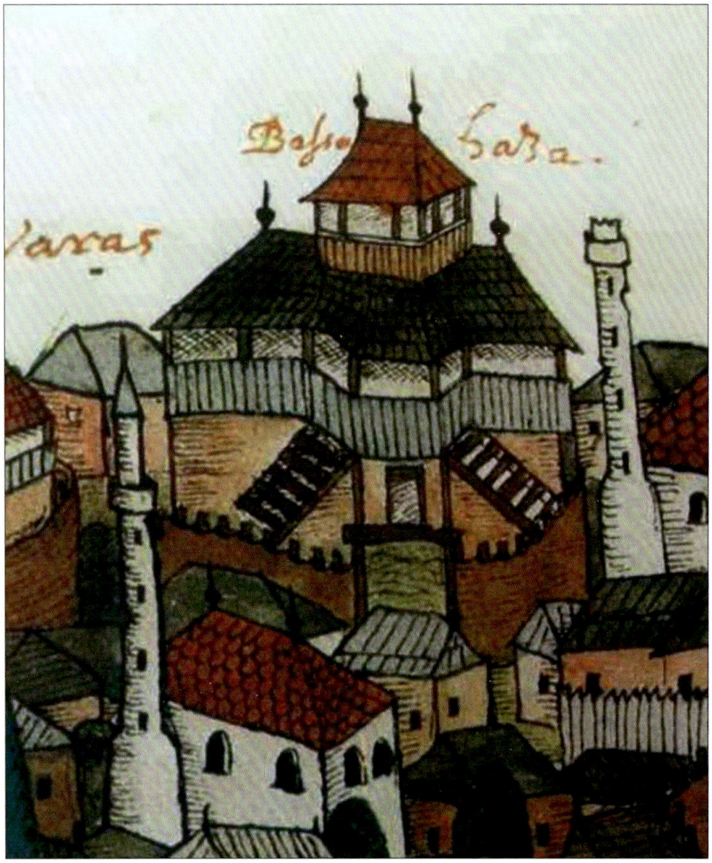

Figure 18. Representation of the Beylerbey's Palace in Timișoara in a drawing by Ferenc Wathay, 1604–1606 (section)

The palace (*saray*) or residence

Ottoman residential buildings had two particularly noteworthy characteristics. One of which was of 'turning inward', which meant that houses would be open and ornamented on the elevations facing the internal courtyard(s) rather than the street. While street elevations would only have small windows, with colonnades leading to the internal courtyards. Houses would usually be several stories high and generally be constructed of wooden frames and adobe bricks. The walls were built on stone foundations. Another characteristic was the use of open spaces. As customary in the Mediterranean region, or perhaps as a throwback to nomadic traditions, rooms were preferred that were open to the outside, with boundaries marked by columns alone (*Figure 18*).

Complexes (*külliye*)

The building types described above would often not stand alone. Wealthy founders would often simultaneously construct a cluster of various buildings with diverse functions in an architecturally homogenous style. The buildings would form a compound that was generally surrounded by boundary wall, the most spectacular example of which is Sultan Süleyman's compound in Istanbul. It included a mosque, a *türbe,* as well as schools and a soup kitchen. All the buildings were incorporated into a single rectangle, with the mosque at the centre (*Figure 19*).

By the 16th and 17th centuries building complexes and groups designed along similar principles appeared throughout the Ottoman Empire, the scale depending on the towns in which they were built, but always significantly smaller than the Sultan's compounds. This was particularly apparent in large cities and in recently occupied towns, where such complexes became symbolic representations of Ottoman power.

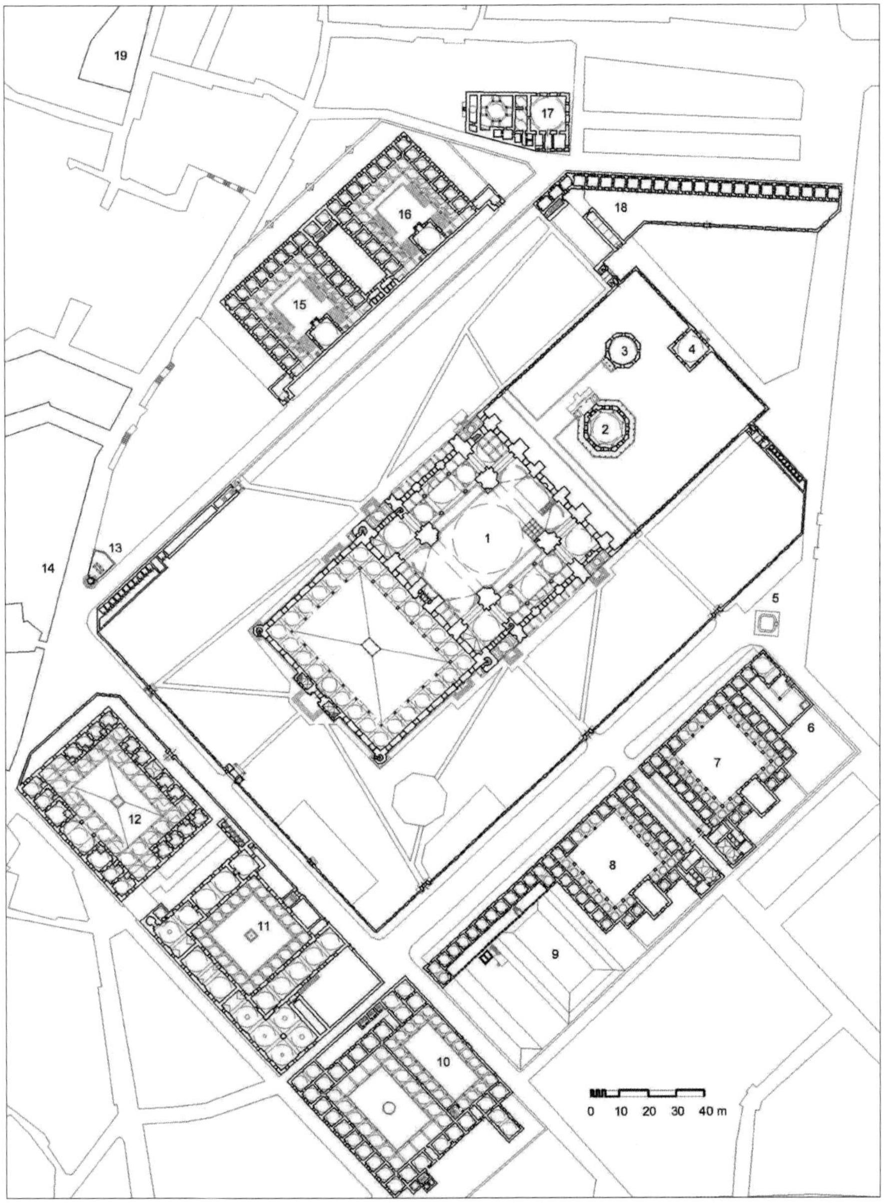

Figure 19. The Süleymaniye complex of buildings (exterior) floorplan, 1550-1557. 1. Mosque. 2. The mausoleum of Süleyman. 3. The mausoleum of Hürrem. 4. Koran recitation school. 5. Public fountain. 6-9., 15-16., 18-19. Schools, various types of madrasa. 9. The remains of a medical school. 10. Infirmary. 11. Poorhouse. 12. Guesthouse. 13. The tomb of Mimar Sinan. 14. Janissary Agha's residence. 17. Baths

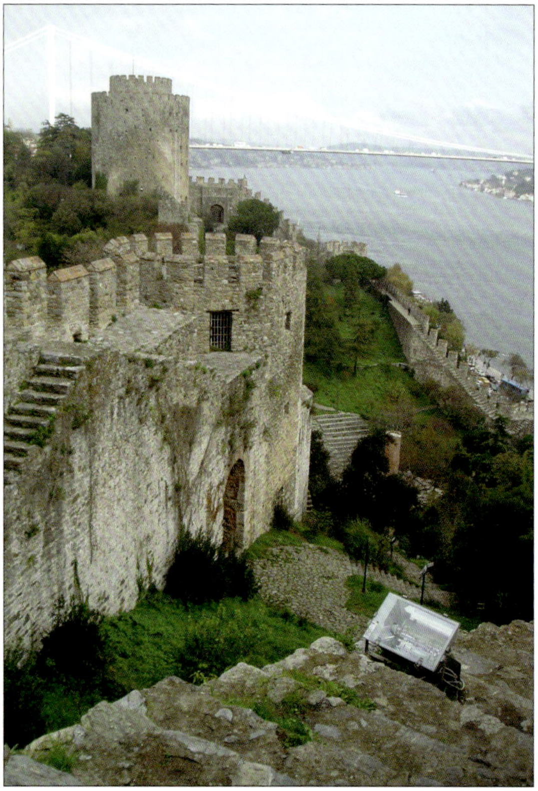

Figure 20. The Rumelian Castle on the banks of the Bosporus in Istanbul, 15th century

Other constructions

In addition, a great many military objects (fortifications, bridges, gunpowder mills) and civilian buildings (such as covered markets), were important means with which the Ottomans consolidated their conquests.

One of Istanbul's most spectacular monuments is the Rumelian Castle (*Figure 20*) that rises from the banks of the Bosphorus. This castle was built by the Turks between 1451-1452 for the siege of Constantinople. It was intended to control traffic on the Bosphorus, and to prevent the city of Constantinople from receiving help during the siege.

During their conquest, the Ottomans encountered innumerable logistical tasks to be resolved. The era's most outstanding engineering achievement was the 28-meter-long Mostar Bridge built over the River Neretva in Bosnia. Sultan Süleyman had given orders for it to be built, but it was only completed after his death. It was blown up during the Balkan War in the 1990s, and the current bridge was rebuilt in the form of the original. We can only wonder at the old bridge in photographs today. Csontváry's famous painting, despite its title The Roman Bridge in Mostar (*Figure 21*), preserves that Ottoman bridge for us.

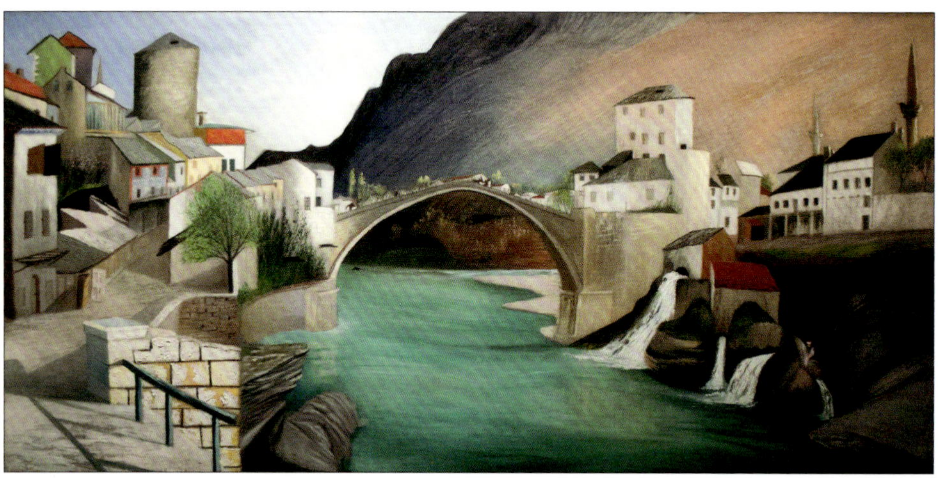

Figure 21. The 16th-century Old Bridge in Mostar, Bosnia. Tivadar Csontváry Kosztka: Roman bridge at Mostar, 1903

IV. Ottoman Architecture in Occupied Hungary

There are still a few cities in Hungary where important Ottoman buildings remain. These buildings stand out in their current urban landscapes. A number of them have survived, but have been overbuilt or reconstructed, with some of the material so concealed that they can only be studied through archaeological methods. Since the conquering Ottomans only settled in strongholds (including walled cities), Ottoman buildings were only ever built in those places. Some fortifications[7] were originally built by the Ottomans, generally earthwork fortifications with wooden structures, known as palankas (palisades), but the brick bastions of Szigetvár were also erected by the Ottomans.[8] Attila Gaál has excavated the wooden Yeni palanka fort (New Palanka)[9] outside Szekszárd, which displays all the characteristics of Ottoman architecture rather well. Remains from the rows of piles that once constituted the fort walls were found, although the original wooden structures had rotted away. The walls of the fort were built by ramming soil between rows of wooden piles. Gyöngyi Kovács[10] has excavated a similar system in Barcs, and Ibolya Gerelyes excavated one in Gyula.[11]

In the case of earlier mediaeval castles, parts previously damaged in battle were repaired, or in some locations, new fortified sections were added. In the northern section of Buda Castle, they raised a new castle wall articulated with fortifications. Excavations extending over several years have been continuously adding detail to our view of the Ottoman construction projects at smaller strongholds such as the one at Csókakő.[12] In Buda, on the northern boundary of the city, a completely separate, smaller fort was built to protect the gunpowder mill (*baruthane*).[13] The mill building, which was used for the manufacture of gunpowder and thus of military importance, was protected by a fort with four corner towers. Construction began under Arslan Pasha, Beylerbey of

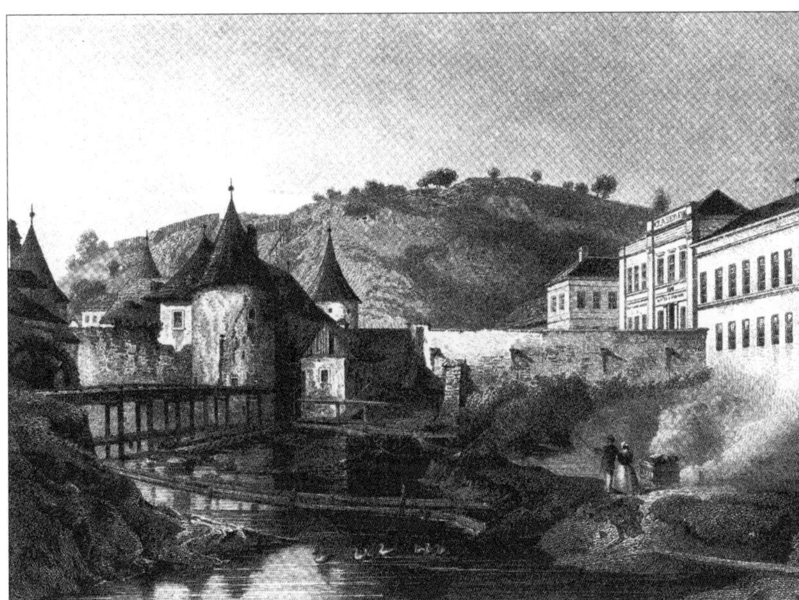

Figure 22. Engraving of the Buda gunpowder mill by Ludwig Rohbock, mid-19th century

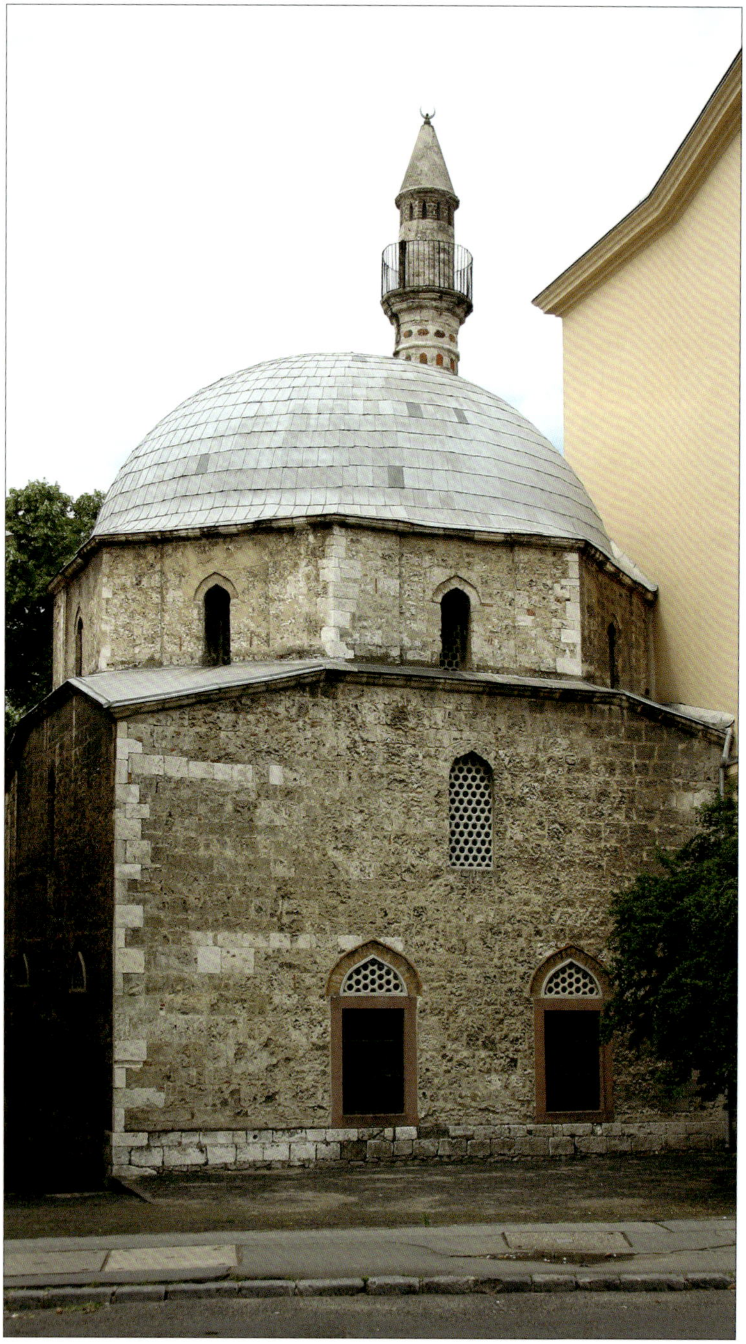

Figure 23. The Yakovali Hasan Pasha Mosque. Pécs, early 17th century

Buda (1565-1566), and was completed by Sokollu Mehmed Pasha (1566-1587) (*Figure 22*).

Along with military construction projects, a significant number of buildings were erected in connection with the cultural and religious systems of institutions of the conquerors. They believed it was very important to facilitate Friday prayers on the very first Friday after any particular settlement was occupied. Since the towns of the mediaeval Hungarian Kingdom they occupied had no mosques, they had to be set up in a matter of days. Following a practice established earlier in the Balkans, they rapidly converted Christian churches: the furniture was removed, the paintings of saints were whitewashed over, any statues were simply walled off or removed, and a *mihrab* niche was cut into the southern wall.[14] The great urgency usually meant that they were usually very simple, lancet-arched niches, such as the one surviving in the Inner City Parish Church of Pest. In the later periods of the conquest–in many cases even in the 16th century–the more powerful pashas and beys built new mosques inside their strongholds,[15] this time in the Ottoman style. Some of the mosques had a square floor plan covered by a dome, there were probably examples constructed in all larger towns, today the most beautiful surviving examples are in Pécs. Ornamental paintings decorated the side walls, still visible at Yakovali Hasan Pasha's mosque in Pécs (*Figure 23-24*). A lobby was usually erected at the entrance, which would be covered by a dome or by a trough vault. However, those building elements were destroyed, and only the foundations of the entrance

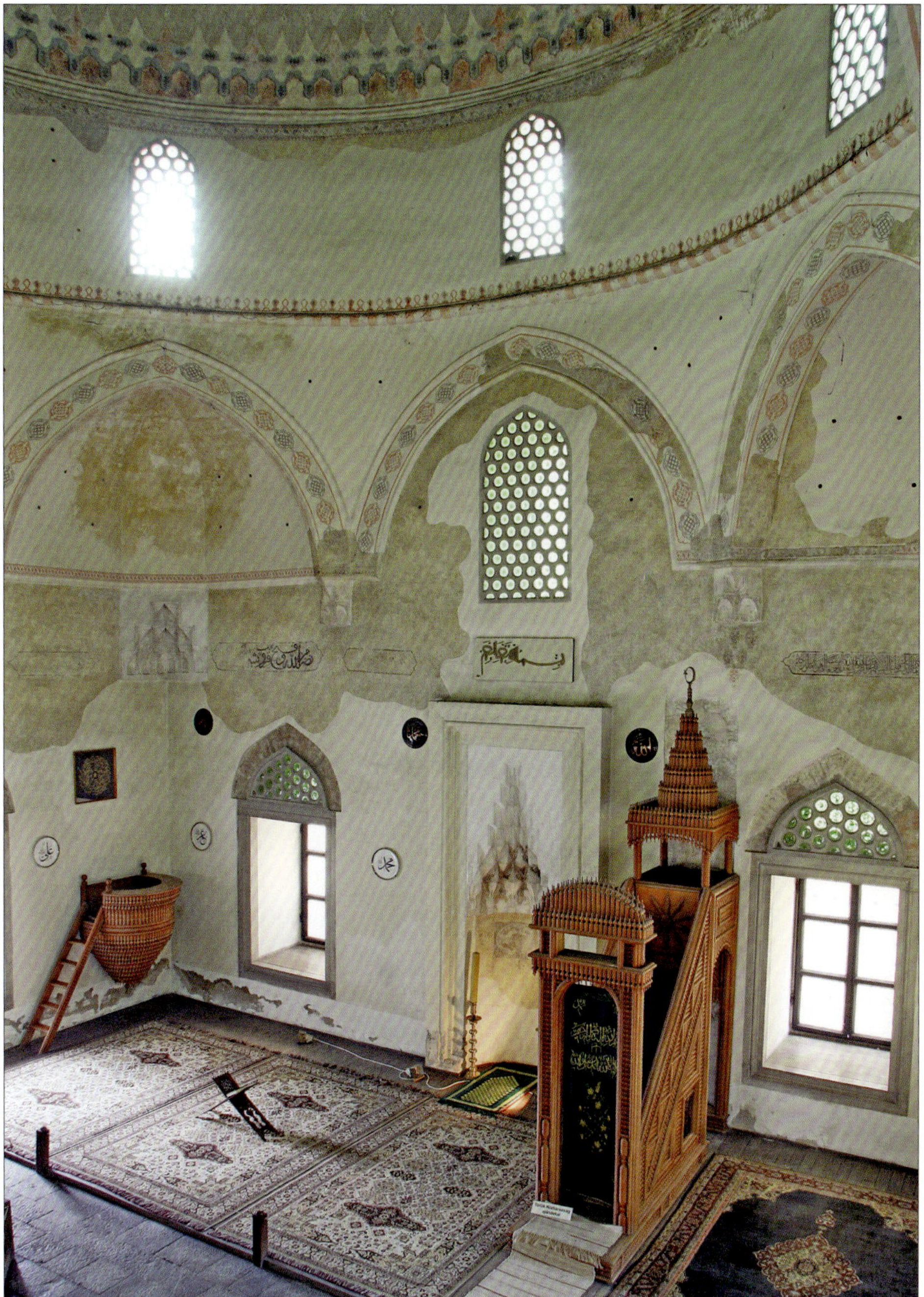

Figure 24. Interior of the Yakovali Hasan Pasha Mosque

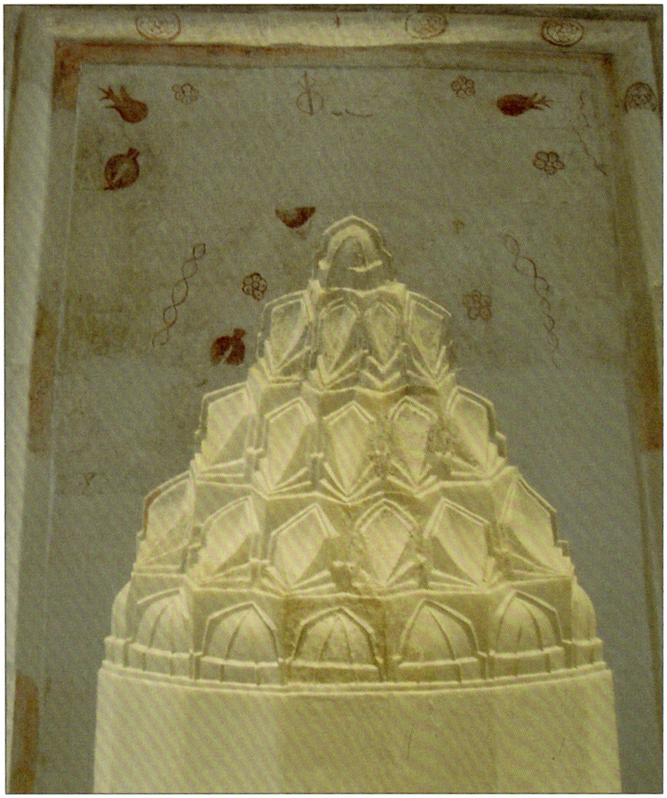

Figure 25. The restored *mihrab* at the Uzicheli Hadji Ibrahim Mosque (early 17th century)

hall at Yakovali Hasan Pasha's mosque remain. Some mosques were built on a rectangular groundplan with flat wooden roofs. Such buildings were preserved in Szigetvár and in Esztergom. The *mihrab* niches in such newly built mosque were much more ornate. The *mihrab* at the Esztergom mosque and its painted ornamentation have been preserved to an extent that merits restoration. The simple but certainly interesting ornamental motifs include the characteristic Ottoman patterns: the tulip and the pomegranate (*Figure 25*). Both ground plans included, alongside the mosque, a characteristically pencil-shaped Ottoman minaret. All in all, the newly built mosques were clearly built in the Ottoman architectural style. The ornamentation of the buildings and the individual architectural components were all executed with the utmost care and professionalism.

As the conquerors settled down, the cults of celebrities who died locally became increasingly important. The 'pilgrimage sites' (*ziyaratgah*), in most cases consisting of an individual tomb, played an important role in that process. The very first one to be built was probably the Gül Baba Türbe[16] that still stands today (*Figure 26*), which was built a few years after the occupation of Buda by the third Beylerbey of Buda, Yahyapashazade Mehmed Pasha (1543-1548). The *türbe* was not a stand-alone building, it belonged to the nearby dervish monastery and is the mausoleum of the first leader of that monastery. Gül Baba must have arrived in Buda with the 1541 campaign, and although legend has it that he died in the siege of Buda, it is more likely that he lived for a few more years in Buda and took an active part in organising the dervish monastery. His mausoleum, in keeping with the Ottoman style of the time, is a small, octagonal stone building covered with a brick dome. The cult of Gül Baba grew gradually as decades passed, and by the 17th century he was considered the patron saint of the city of Buda. His cult spread and survived around the Balkans, too, and even today pilgrims come to visit his grave. Although less well known, Idris Baba's mausoleum also survives, in Pécs (*Figure 27*).[17] Like so many other *türbes*,[18] destruction was the fate of the mausoleum built outside Szigetvár for Sultan Süleyman who had died during the siege of the town, where the heart of the monarch was buried.[19] Süleyman's body was taken to Istanbul where his mausoleum forms part of the Süleymaniye complex. The foundations of his *türbe* at Szigetvár, and also the mosque and the dervish monastery built alongside it were recently discovered.[20] A period ground plan for the complex built around the *türbe* and the stronghold has survived in a drawing produced in 1664 by the palatine Pál Eszterházy. The *türbe* of Sokollu Mustafa, Beylerbey of Buda, has also been destroyed, but we know that it was located in Buda and was attributed to Mimar Sinan. The strength of the pasha's family ties–his uncle was the grand vizier–were such that his mausoleum was designed by none other than the chief architect of the empire. The significance of that fact increases still further if we consider that of the 45 *türbes* that Sinan designed in total, only five were built outside Istanbul, including the one in Buda.[21]

As for the Ottoman residences, barely a trace was left of those buildings, archaeology and written sources provide the information we have about them. Many travellers visited Buda during the Ottoman occupation, and the most informative descriptions were provided by a 16th-century trader and diplomat Hans Dernschwam.[22] His experience is particularly important because he had already visited Buda prior to the occupation, so he had seen the city when it was still a royal seat. A few decades later he returned to what had become the capital and hub of an Ottoman

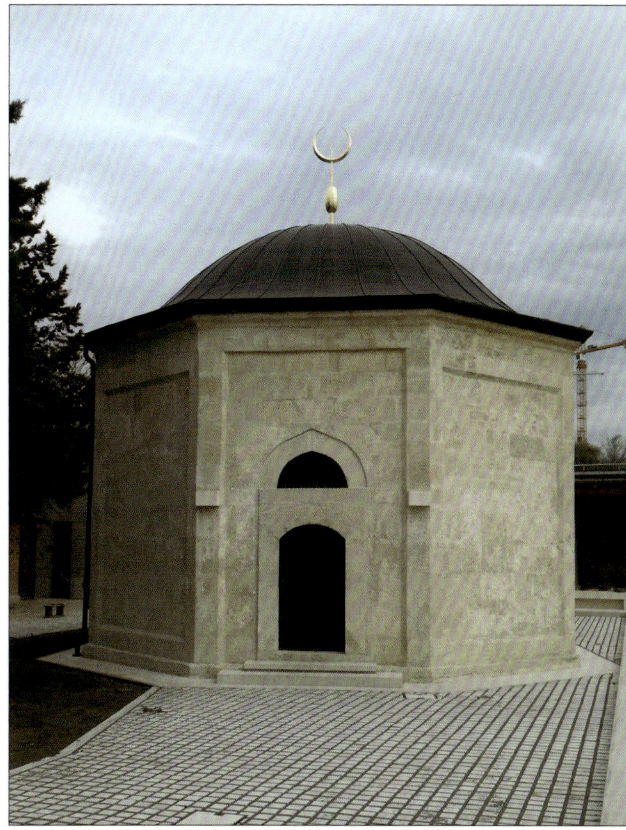

Figure 26. The mausoleum of Gül Baba in Buda, 1543-1548

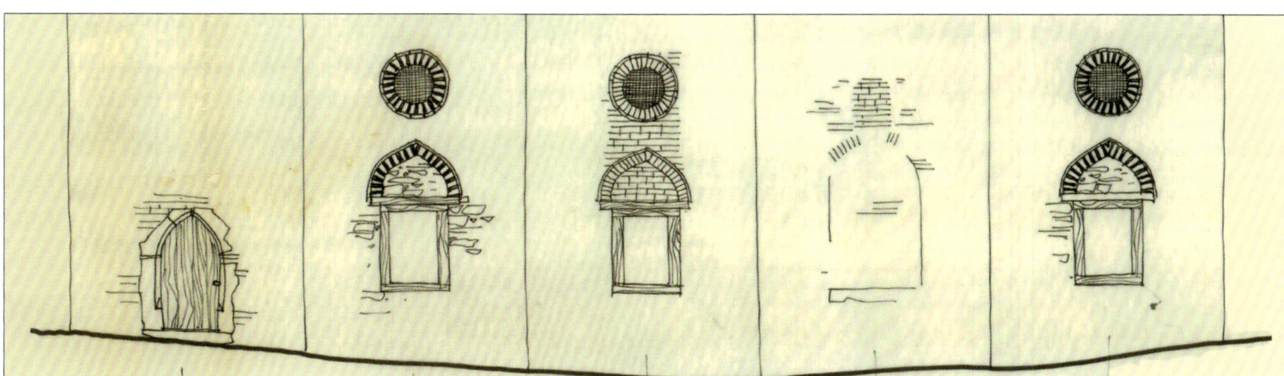

Figure 27. The exterior façade of the mausoleum of Idris Baba (end of the 16th century) on the 1961 restoration plans of Károly Ferenczy (section)

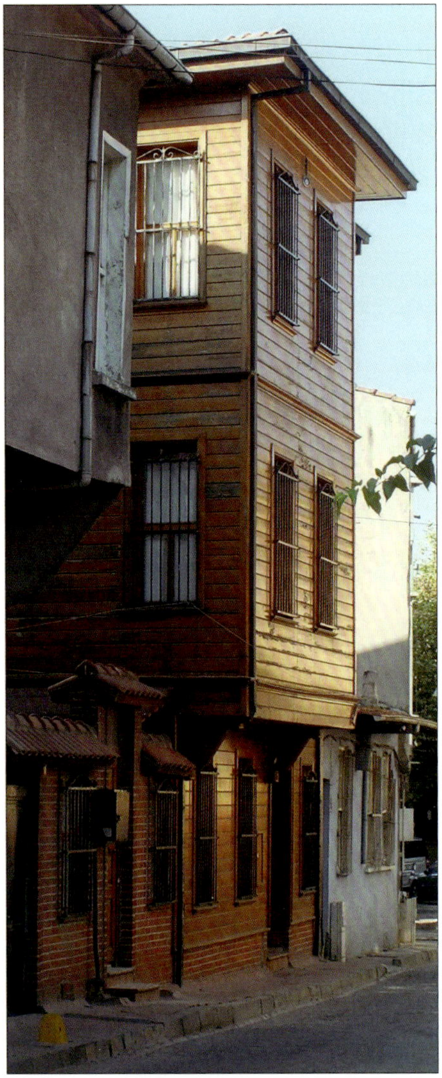

Figure 28. Wooden building structure in today's Istanbul

province, and the changes he observed were striking: the once sparkling, royal city had become a dilapidated, ramshackle settlement. Dernschwam writes of boarded up windows and walls made of mud. Almost a hundred years later the Ottoman traveller Evliya Çelebi[23] reported a beautiful city. Who was correct? In actual fact, they were both right. The Buda described by Dernschwam and then by Evliya are one and the same in all respects except they were viewed from different cultural perspectives. Dernschwam was accustomed to Western norms and architectural principles, so his eyes detected a city in a state of decrepitude, where the once beautiful Renaissance and Gothic buildings had been spoiled with walled-up windows, and extensions to existing buildings built from adobe bricks. From another perspective, the conquering Ottomans were simply attempting to make this mediaeval city conform more to their own requirements and their own architectural norms. The street elevations of Ottoman houses are small and have few windows; however, as we have already mentioned, their porches and windows tended to face inwards towards the courtyards, which is why the windows on the street elevations of Buda houses were walled up. Artisans tended to live alongside their workshops, which, being open towards the street, were furnished by adding small extensions to the houses on the street side. As a result, the narrow streets typical of Eastern cities appeared in Buda, too. The extensions were built according to Ottoman custom: a stone foundation was first built on which a wooden frame formed the structural component of walls, and the spaces between the beams were filled with adobe bricks. The same technique was also used to build all new residences, even the palaces of the Beylerbeys of Buda.[24] What Dernschwam actually saw in the city was not poverty, but the imprint of a totally alien way of construction, precisely the reason Evliya Chelebi found the city so familiar and beautiful (*Figure 28*).

One interesting and noteworthy example of Ottoman architecture in Hungary is furnished by the bridge over the River Tisza at Szolnok. While the large quantities of wood used in wooden forts perished completely over the centuries, several dozen wooden piles from the wooden Ottoman bridge remain. In one dry year, the water of the Tisza fell so low that the ends of the piles stuck out of the water. After a natural historical study, the research clearly identified the structure as an Ottoman bridge.[25] Another special complex of finds associated with Ottoman bridge-building is located in the bed of the River Dráva: the remains of a short-lived pontoon bridge at Drávatamási (so-called 'tree-trunk boats') have been documented in archaeological research.[26]

V. The General Characteristics of Turkish Baths

Ottoman bath architecture reaches back to the bath architecture of earlier Islamic empires, which in turn derived from the Roman tradition. Roman baths did not fully meet the requirements of Islamic culture and religion, so the system of buildings underwent alteration. For muslims, it was important to bathe in running water, so the old pools were slowly removed from the baths to be replaced by wall fountains. In the early buildings of Islam—for example, in the baths at the 8th-century desert palace of Qusair Amra (Jordan)—we still see pools and even walls adorned by frescoes. The Seljuk Turks established their characteristic architectural style in the 11th to 13th centuries,[27] and the ground plans that were later characteristic of Ottoman bath architecture were already in evidence there. Consequently, those buildings can be considered the immediate precursors to Ottoman baths.

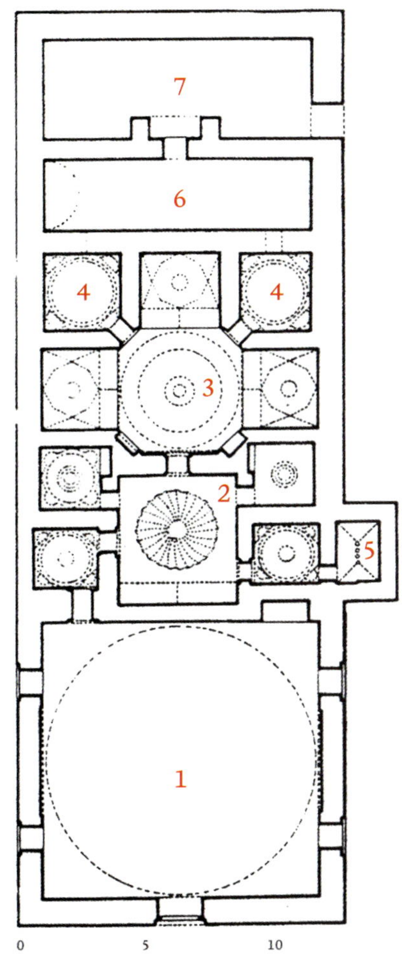

Figure 29. Groundplan of the steam baths, Sultan Emir Baths, Bursa, 1426. 1. Entrance hall. 2. Warm room. 3. Hot room. 4. Private baths. 5. Toilet. 6. Cistern. 7. Heating room

The layout of Ottoman baths

Ottoman baths have three main sections: the entrance hall (*jamakhan* or *soyunmalik*), the warm room(s) (*iliklik*) and the hot room (*harara* or *sijaklik*) (*Figure 29*). The entrance hall was usually the largest room, a sizeable square room where patrons could change. An ornamental fountain was placed at the centre and benches around the sides. In most cases, a number of smaller square or rectangular halls opened off the entrance hall, these were the warm rooms. Their walls were also lined with stone benches and wall fountains. Those rooms were kept warm using underfloor heating and, given their distance from the boiler room, the temperature was never too high. The innermost space of the baths was the hot room, which was directly adjacent to the boiler room and the hot water tank, so it was extremely hot. It was usually larger than the warm room(s), and its layout followed strict convention. The middle of the room was occupied by the usually octagonal 'navel stone' (*göbek tashi*), and stone benches lined the walls upon which wall fountains were placed. The water lines have taps fixed to the walls, with small, marble basins underneath (*kurna*).

The rooms listed were always present, even in small baths. The large baths differed in the sizes of the individual rooms and in that they had more warm rooms, additionally, alongside the hot rooms, they also had private baths (*halvet*). Adjacent to the rooms frequented by patrons, there were a series of rooms for water treatment and heating where large, walled up water cisterns, a boiler room and the wood storage facility were all located. All of the baths also had toilets, generally near the warm rooms.

Steam baths - thermal baths

Ottoman steam baths usually utilised water from rivers, streams or wells. The water was collected in the above-mentioned large cisterns built alongside the baths and warmed using a fire made in the furnace room on the floor below. Hot air was conducted into the floor heating system under the baths' rooms, thereby heating the building. Hot water and cold water were kept in separate reservoirs were delivered to the wall fountains along ceramic water conduits built into the walls. These steam baths were known as *hamams*, originally an Arabic term (*Figure 30*).

The Ottomans also made use of hot springs. Wherever those were found, baths with a somewhat different structure were built. There was no need for a furnace because the thermal water from the hot spring was sufficiently hot already. The thermal springs had added benefits as well, for instance they had very high yields and therapeutic effects. Thermal baths also had pools built, in most cases just the one, but rarely two or even three. The large surface area of hot water took care of heating the building, so the floor heating system could also be dispensed with. Apart from that, the tripartite articulation (entrance hall - warm room - hot room) was still in evidence, and the appearance of the buildings was also very similar to steam baths. In Turkish, thermal baths are called *ilija* or *kaplija* (*Figure 31*).

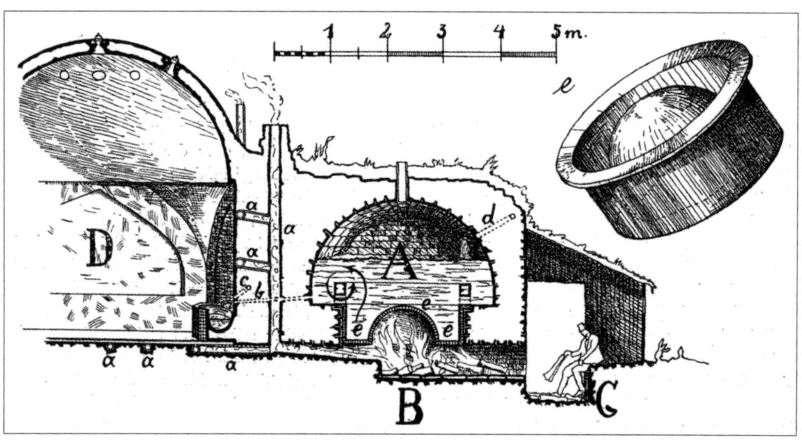

Figure 30. Diagram of the steam bath heating system.
A. Built cistern. B. Fireplace.
C. Heating room. D. Bathing area

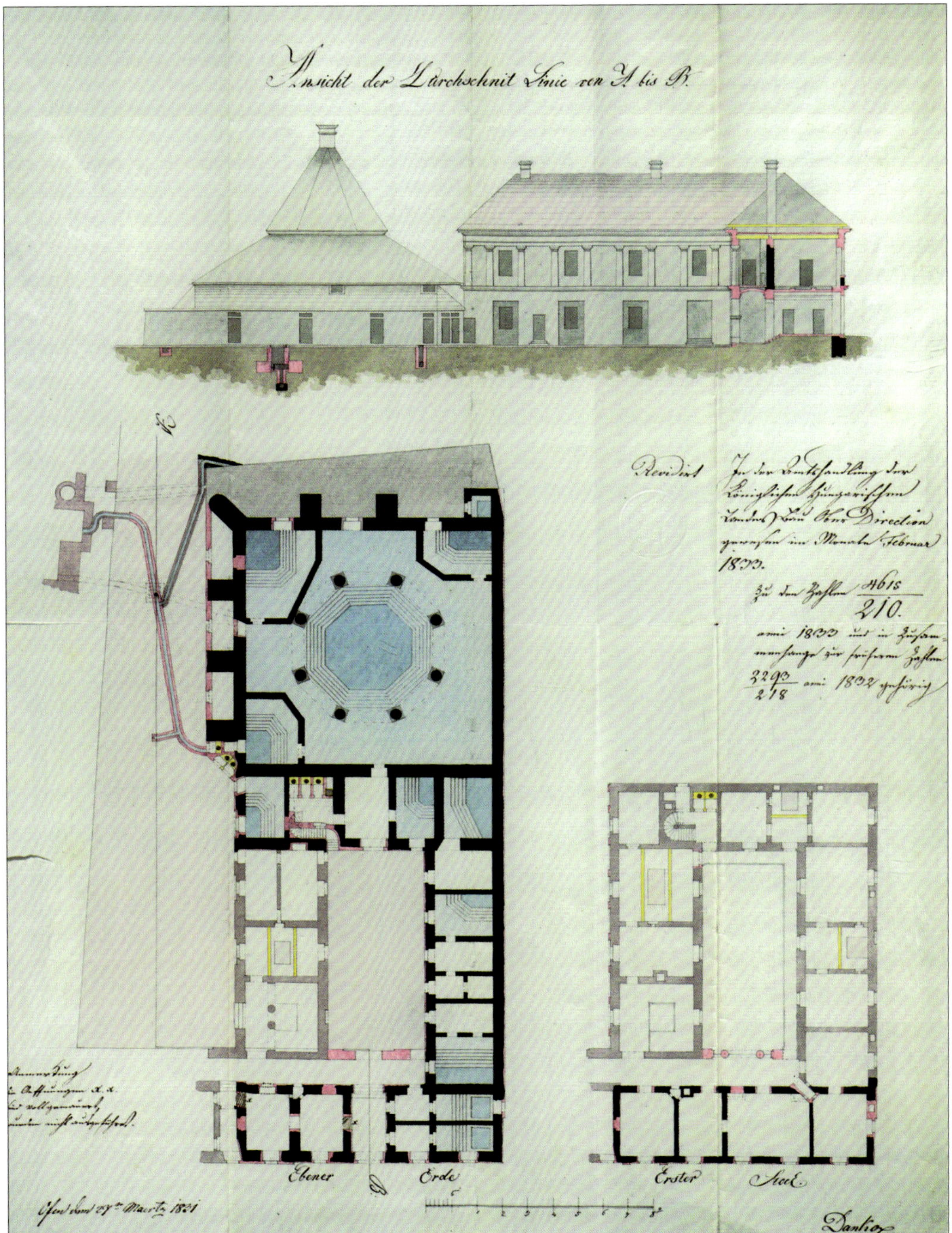

Figure 31. A floorplan of the Rudas Baths from a survey made in 1833 (József Dankó's plan)

As thermal springs are quite rare, the number of thermal baths built around the empire was much lower than that of steam baths, although there were many in cities with thermal springs. On the other hand, steam baths were built in every corner of the empire, even in smaller towns.

Public baths - private baths

The majority of the baths were open to all for a relatively low fee. They were usually founded and owned by the Sultan (the state) and members of the Ottoman elite, or charitable foundations (*vakf*) that they established. Accordingly, public baths were usually not stand-alone buildings, but formed parts of building complexes (*külliye*). There were often markets, a mosque, a caravanserai or a pilgrimage site and so on, nearby.

Baths were also built inside palaces, summer and winter residences and monasteries, but they were only for the use of the community in question. These private baths were smaller than the public ones, sometimes consisting of only two rooms, an antechamber and a hot room.

Double baths

At any particular time, baths could only be used by either women or men, therefore days were divided between the sexes. However, there existed a solution for allowing both sexes to use the baths at the same time: they simply built two very similar buildings side by side, but separated (*Figure 32*). One half of the double baths catered to women, the other half to men. Both baths had their own entrance halls, warm rooms and hot room, but the men's section was usually larger and more ornate, and it opened into the busier street. The women's section was usually more modest and opened from a side street. Builders liked this solution, partly perhaps because the two separate parts could be served by a single water management system. About a third of all baths were double baths of that type.

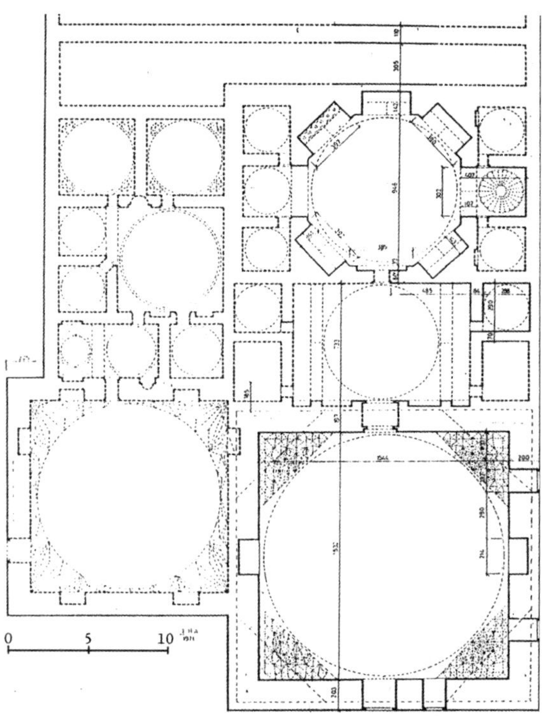

Figure 32. Floorplan of the double baths, clearly showing they were built alongside each other. Tahtakale Baths, Istanbul, 15th century

The types of baths according to their architectural layouts

As we have seen, the rooms of the baths follow each other in strict sequence, partly due to technical requirements and partly to custom. The bath-houses, which are all very similar in their floor plans, yet differ in the most striking manner in accordance with the solutions used to maintain their hot rooms. It is, therefore, customary to classify such buildings in accordance with those solutions.[28] The types established by Turkish researchers must be extended on the basis of our experience in Hungary, resulting in a total of eight different bath-house floor plans (*Figure 33*).

A/ Cross-shaped hot room with four *eyvans*, with private baths on the corners. The corners of the large, square room have smaller square rooms built inside them (private baths). The corner rooms and the centre of the hot room are covered with domes, while the area between the centre and the corner room is barrel vaulted or has trough vaults. It has versions with two, three or four eyvans.

B/ Star-shaped hot room: From the outside, this building stands on a square base, but inside it forms an octagonal room the sides of which contain large wall-niches. The central part is covered with a dome.

C/ Square hot room with little private baths arranged around it: two or three sides of the square hot room are lined by square private baths of various dimensions. Each one of those has a dome of its own. This is a rare, archaic layout.

D/ Multi-domed type: the hot room is divided into identical sections by vaults, and the individual sections are covered by domes of identical size.

E/ The central dome type, has a broad hot room and double private baths: the square ground plan is divided in half across, the front room is the hot room, an elongated rectangle, the middle part is has a dome over it, the two side sections have some other roof. The passage to the two small rooms, also covered with separate domes and built next to the hot room (the private baths) opens from beneath the central dome. The floor plan of the hot room and the two smaller rooms together forms a square.

F/ This type is topped with identical domes: it was a solution generally used in smaller baths: the warm and the hot room, and the one or more private baths were all identical in size. Each one has its personal dome.

G/ The Colonnade type: the dome above the centre of the hot room is supported by columns, there are barrel vaults in the spaces between the dome and the side walls.

H/ The single dome type: usually square or, less frequently, octagonal hall, with no further articulation of the floor plan, and with no private baths adjoining it. A typical arrangement for small baths.

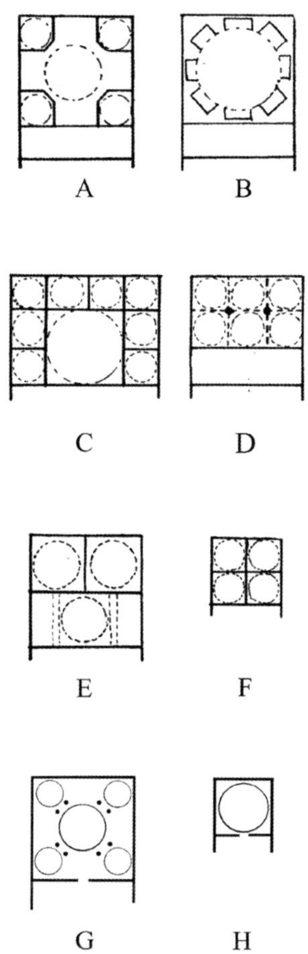

Figure 33. A typological division based on the layout of the hot room, based on Semavi Eyice's typology

Open baths - baths in buildings

Bathing was permitted not only in the fine, purpose-built baths described above.[29] The contemporary descriptions of Buda also mention examples of 'open' (*achik*) and 'timber' (*tahtali*) baths. Near the northern and southern thermal springs of Buda, there were lakes, which were also used for bathing. In 19th-century Istanbul, an area of water was walled off for bathing at the end of a pier extending into the sea[30] (*Figure 34*). Similar structures may have been built on the shores of Hungarian lakes during the 16th and 17th centuries.

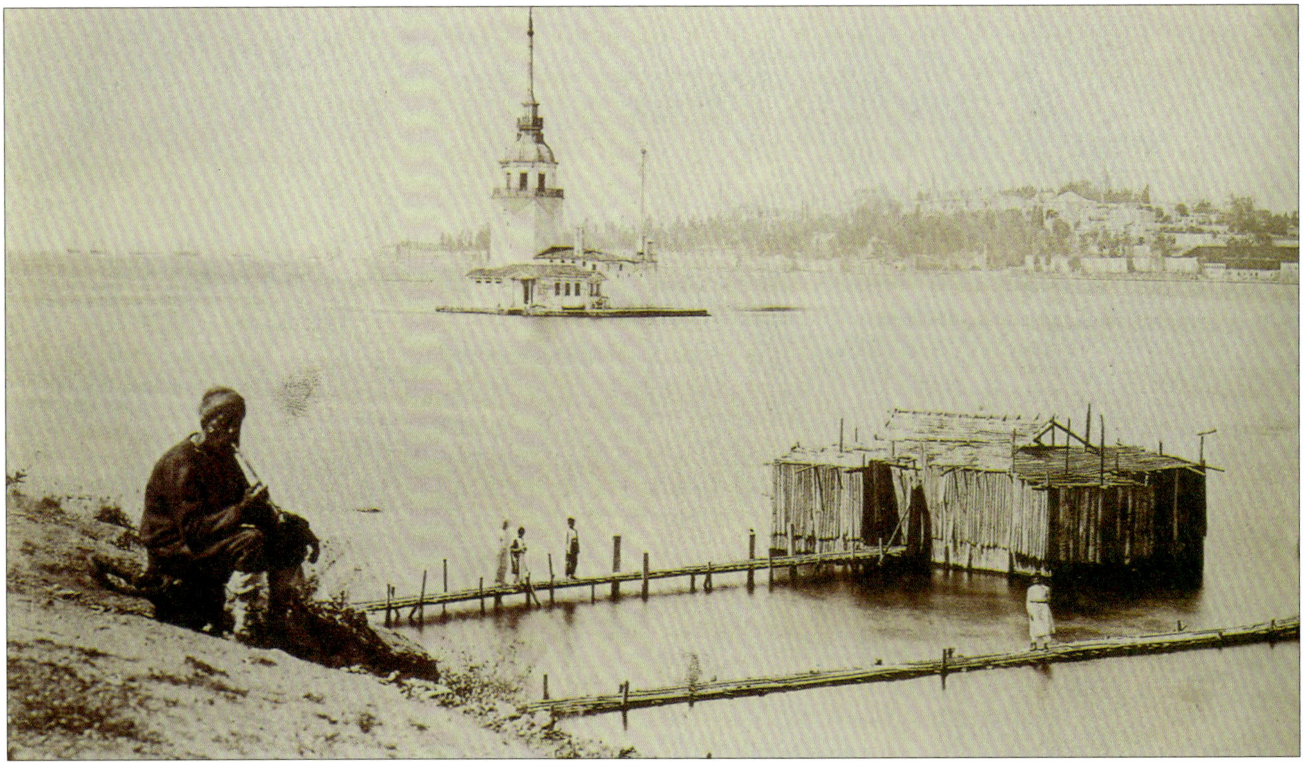

Figure 34. Seawater baths in Istanbul in the 19th century

The appearance of classical Ottoman era baths

The great majority of the Turkish baths in Hungary were built in the 16th century, shortly after the respective towns were conquered by the Ottomans. This was the classical era of Ottoman architecture, and the greatest architect of the day was Mimar Sinan, discussed above. Although by that time, Ottoman architectural style had fully developed its formal characteristics, in all probability Sinan personally contributed to the similarities between individual functional building types.

This was also true of the baths that were built in the 16th century. The floor plans of those buildings generally fit into a single large rectangle, half of which is occupied by the large entrance hall, the other half by the hot room, with warm rooms lined up in the space left between them. The rooms were arranged along an axis with the entrance in the middle of the elevation, opening via a door onto a warm room, followed by another door leading to the hot room. Among the ground floor variations of the hot rooms, the most popular was the cross-shaped room (A type), followed by the double private bath layout (E). It was a high-profile change from the baths of earlier periods (*Figures 35-36*) that

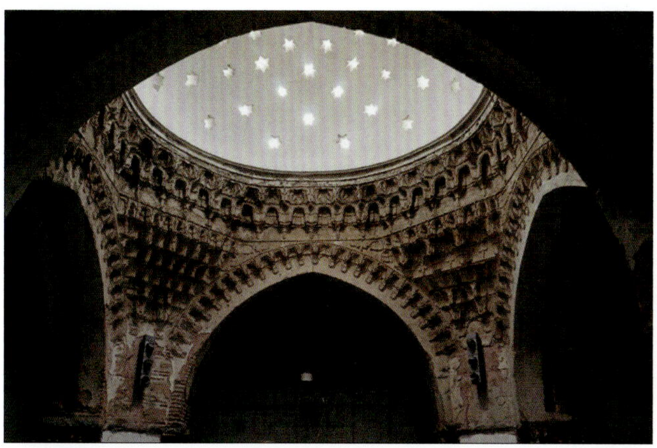

Figure 35. The dome of the Davut Pasha Baths in Skopje, 1489-1497

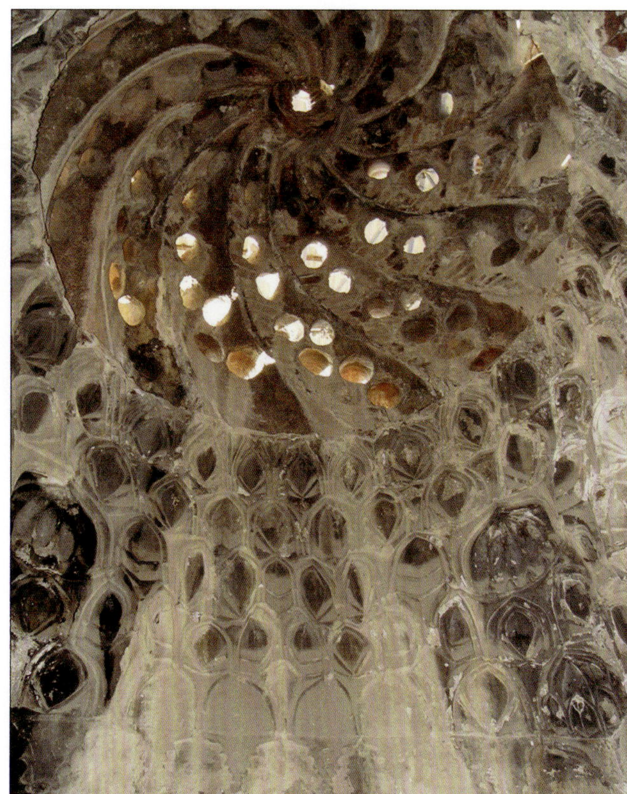

Figure 36. The ornate dome of the Ismail Bey Baths in Iznik, 14th century

significantly less effort was expended in ornamenting the building: the bulbous, stalactite-like lobes that had once covered almost the entire inner surface of domes and vaults now disappeared; they began to be replaced by smaller versions of these plastic ornaments placed in corners, fashioned from stone or plaster and reminiscent of stalactites. It was Sinan himself who introduced some personal variation to the relatively strict principles of architecture. His work is characterised by many minor details that make the buildings that he personally designed stand out from the rest. The composition of the Istanbul steam bath of Sultan Hürrem (*Figure 37*) is a rare solution with the two parts of the double baths one placed behind the other. The layout of the colonnaded space outside the entrance hall and the changes in the shapes of the auxiliary spaces–e.g. in the steam bath known as the Sokollu Mehmed Pasha Baths in Istanbul, or the steam bath of Sultan Atik Valide–the construction of a colonnaded hot room and the attachment of auxiliary spaces to the exterior walls of the buildings were all novel ideas dreamed up by Sinan.[31]

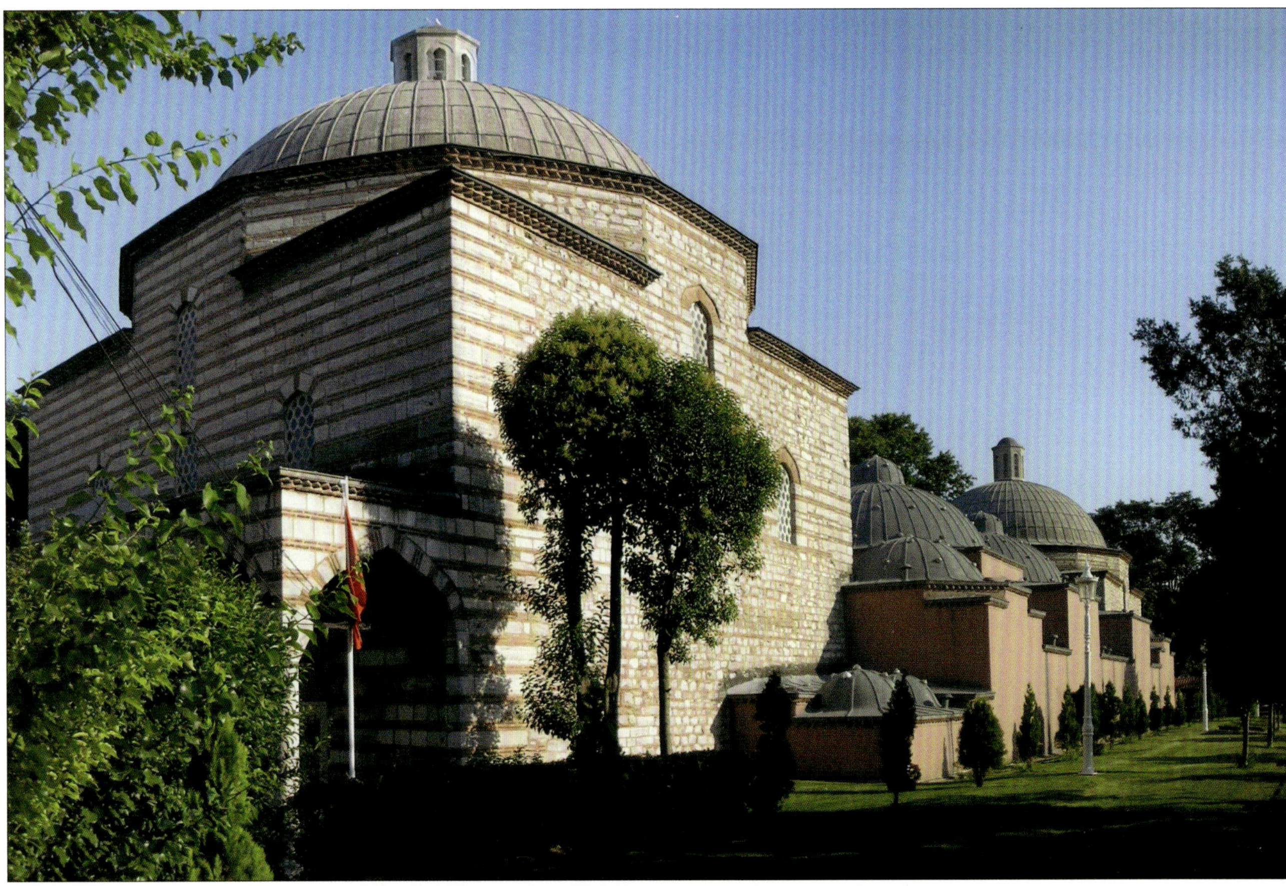

Figure 37. The Sultan Hürrem Baths in Istanbul, 16th century

VI. The Use of Turkish Baths

There were no residential bathrooms at that time, so the primary purpose of Turkish baths was personal hygiene. People seeking health cures also frequented thermal waters, aware of the health benefits. Furthermore, the baths were also an important social venue, particularly for women, for whom it was practically the only place where they could meet without being accompanied by men. In the lives of high-born women, who were almost never allowed out of the section of their houses for females, going to the baths was a particularly important event.

How were baths used in the 16th and 17th centuries? Guests changed in the entrance hall, leaving their shoes under the stone benches that lined the walls and their clothing in wall niches. The bench had rush matting or carpets on it, where guests could sit down for a chat, to rest, or drink coffee or even smoke a pipe. They left the very hot inner rooms and came to the entrance hall to cool down before returning to the hot room again. Somewhere near the entrance, the bath servant sat, and collected entrance fees. Extra services, such a massages and depilation, were charged separately.

Some estate records also list the objects that guests took to the baths with them: they included the small brass bowl that people used douse themselves, bath shirts and bathing gloves.[32] They received large towels at the baths. Although not yet apparent in 16th-century miniatures, slippers can also be seen in 18th and 19th century depictions (*Figure 38*). The floor heating system that kept the rest of the baths warm did not extend beneath the entrance hall. In colder climates, in winter, a *mangal*, a charcoal-burning heater made of brass was used for heating, or an open fireplace was built into one of the walls.

Once guests had changed, they entered the warm section. In larger baths, there would be a number of smaller rooms arranged between the entrance hall and the hot rooms, which were all pleasantly warm. That's where people cleaned themselves, and where depilation was also performed, amongst other services. During the 16th and 17th century, men usually also had all the hair removed from their bodies (except their heads). The operation was performed by bath servants. Hot and cold water was available from the wall fountains along the walls. The water ran onto the floor, where drains were built to carry the dirty water away towards the toilets.

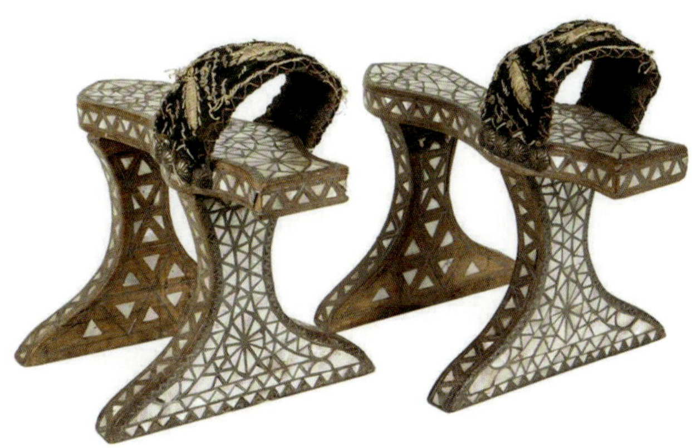

Figure 38. Bath slippers, late 19th - early 20th century

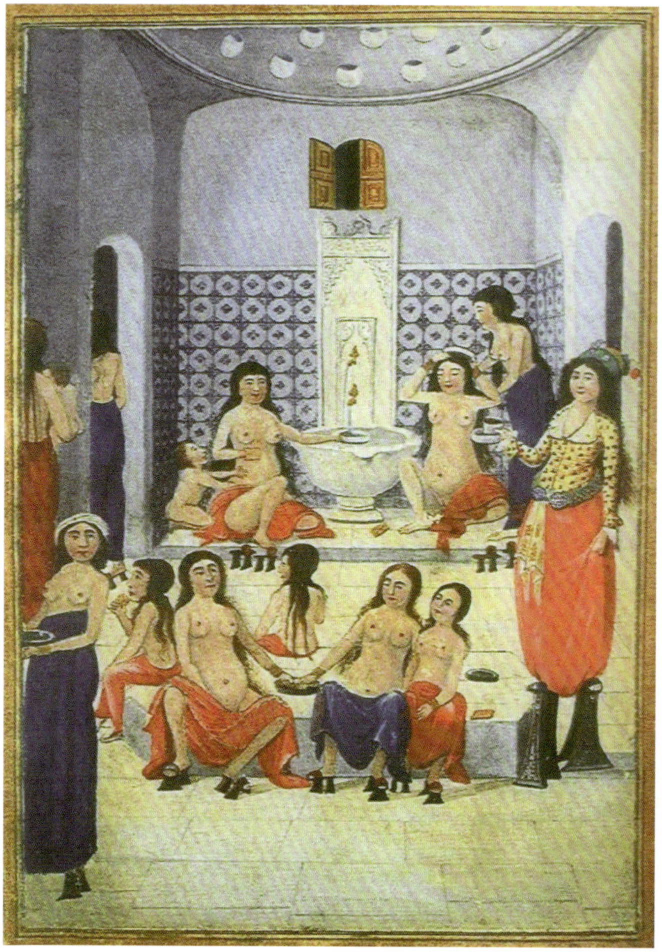

Figure 39. Bathing woman in an 18th-century depiction

The innermost room of the baths was the hot room, the use of which was fundamentally different in steam baths and in thermal baths. The centre of the hot rooms of thermal baths was occupied by a large pool filled with medicinal water that was also used for its therapeutic effects. As with today's medicinal baths, guests would sit for specific periods of time on the number of occasions prescribed for their treatment (*Figure 39*). The miniatures also show some swimmers,[33] although the shallow pools, which were only about one metre deep, offered little opportunity to swim. The hot rooms of steam baths, on the other hand, was occupied by the navel-stone which, despite its name, was not a single large piece of stone, but a constructed pedestal. Guests could sit or lie on it, have the bath servants give them a massage or attend to their personal hygiene. Both types of baths had benches along the walls, with wall fountains for washing. Guests sat on the stone bench and let some water into the marble basins of the fountains. The water running onto the floor was gathered into a gutter under the floor. Along the wall, there would be occasional larger blocks of stone, which were used for seating older or ill people for whom the stone benches were too low.

The private bath (or private baths) opened from the hot room. Those allowed four or five people, usually relatives or friends, to have a bath together, privately. When one of those private baths was in use, a curtain was drawn across its entrance to indicate that it was occupied. The layout of those small rooms was identical to all the others with running water: there was a stone bench around the edges, with wall fountains on it. In some thermal baths, the private baths had their own little pools.

The baths were cleaned daily and regularly maintained. Particular care was taken at thermal baths, where the water in the pools was replaced daily.

VII. Turkish Baths in Hungary

At one point in time the region of today's Hungary had at least forty-six baths, the number about which we have written records.[34] Only sixteen of those, however, are preserved today to any extent: they will be described in detail in the chapter on individual baths. Some buildings are still almost intact, while only the foundation walls have been found of others. There are written sources that tell us about the people who founded the baths, sometimes telling about their positions, their name, and in a few cases travellers have even furnished us with illustrative descriptions of them. All that knowledge has been supplemented by the surviving maps and floor plans.

Written sources mention baths in twenty-nine fortified towns (*Figure 40*). In most of those towns, there was a single Turkish bath, but some larger cities had several: Buda had seven, while Eger, Esztergom, Székesfehérvár, Pest and Pécs

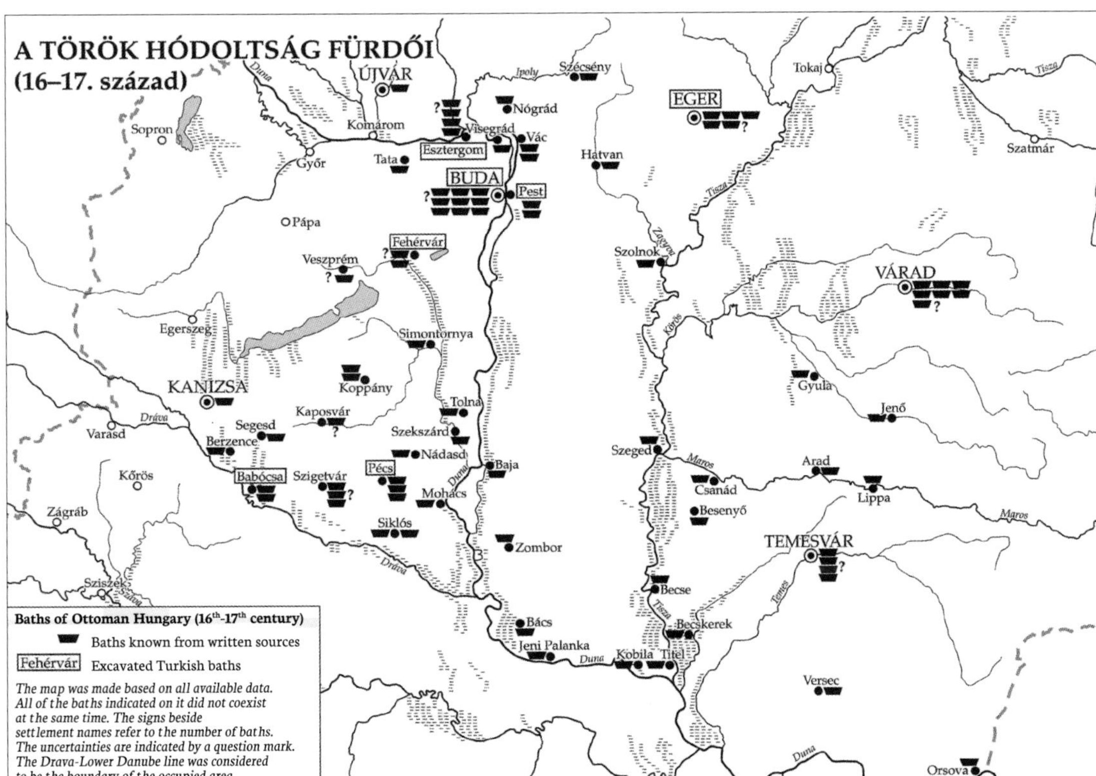

Figure 40. Turkish baths in Ottoman Hungary

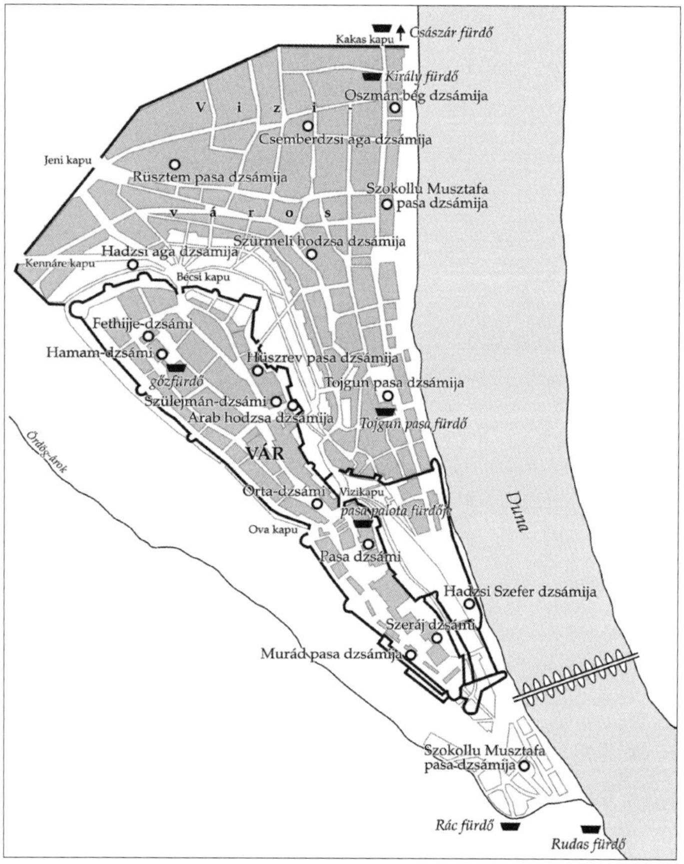

Figure 41. Turkish baths in Buda

had two or three each. In Buda, there were six public baths, of which four were thermal (today's Császár, Király, Rác and Rudas baths), while the other two were steam baths (one of which, the Toygun Pasha, was a double structure (*Figure 41*). There was also a private bath at the palace of the Buda beylerbeys on Castle Hill. In addition to the constructed baths, the natural thermal water lakes of the northern and the southern group of springs also attracted a number of open baths, which, however, were probably more like today's beaches, or outdoor pools. The exact locations of the baths have primarily been taken from a 1686 map produced by Marcell de la Vigne[35] and from a number of panoramic images. The contemporary names were preserved in the writings of travellers[36] and in the inventories that were taken after the city was reoccupied.[37]

The first one of the baths to be completed was the steam baths on Castle Hill, whose archaeological remains, however, have never been found. Later, Toygun, the Beylerbey of Buda built his mosque and next to it his baths in Víziváros, in the early 1550's. The four thermal baths in Buda were associated with the rule of Sokollu Mehmed Pasha (1566-1578), who purchased the Rác Baths (known as the Little Baths or the Tabán Baths during the Ottoman era) and had the other three built: the Rudas Baths, the Király Baths and the Császár Baths (contemporaneously known respectively as the 'Green Pillar Baths', the 'Cockerel Gate Baths' and the 'Veli Bey Baths'. The city's seventh baths were the only known private baths[38] and were located in the palace of the Buda beylerbeys, built on Castle Hill during the Fifteen Years War. Six of those seven baths are also known to archaeology; indeed, the four thermal baths have been in continuous operation since their foundation.

Three baths were built in Pécs, all three steam baths. Two of those—Memi Pasha's and Ferhad Pasha's—were double baths (*Figure 42*). Thanks to a survey produced by Joseph de Haüy, we know the precise location of each of them. The imperial military engineer (who had also worked in Buda) produced his map in 1687 following the battles of the re-conquest. The remnants of Memi Pasha's Baths were excavated next to today's Saint Francis Church by Győző Gerő.[39] With

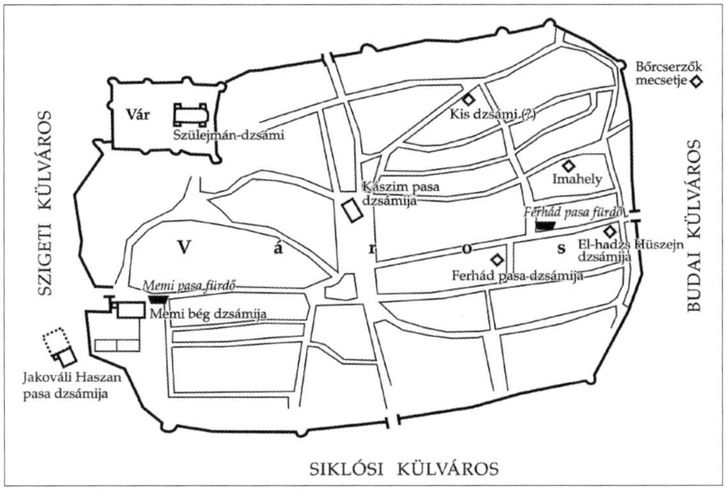

Figure 42. Excavation of the Turkish baths in Pécs

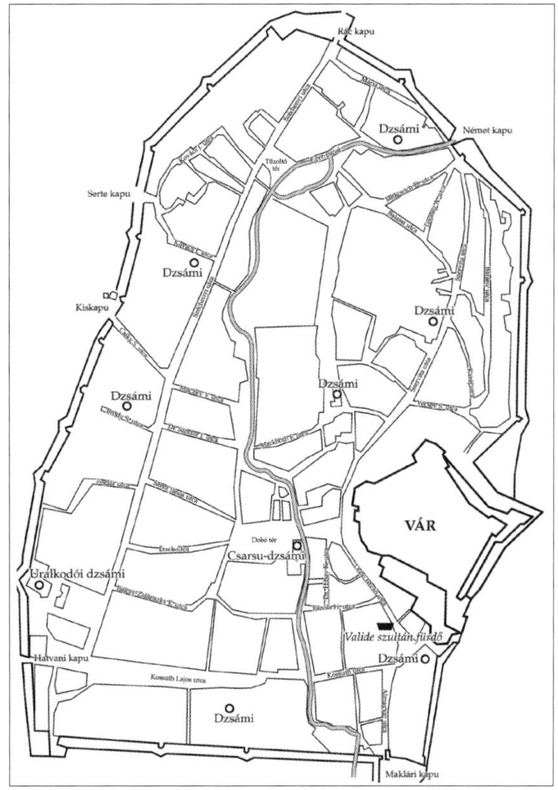

Figure 43. Excavation of the Turkish baths in Eger

regards to Ferhad Pasha's Baths, a detailed architectural survey has survived from the 18th century[40] and the site underwent archaeological excavation in 1984. Kasim Pasha's Baths stood near his mosque, in the north-eastern corner of the main square, its archaeological remains have never been found. Written sources from the middle of the 16th century also mention a state-owned steam baths, but it is unclear whether that was in fact identical to any of the three baths mentioned above.[41]

Evliya Chelebi wrote about two steam baths in Eger (*Figure 43*), although he did note that the thermal springs of the town were not as beautifully cultivated as those in Buda. One of the baths, that of the Valide Sultan, that is the 'baths of the sultan's mother' (*Valide Sultan Hamami*) is well known from archaeological surveys, but the other is a moot point.[42] The thermal baths in the town on the shore of the Eger Stream are still in use today, which may well have had an Ottoman precursor, as its octagonal, domed hall is characteristically reminiscent of Ottoman baths. But research on the building has not yet determined its origins. Some of the solutions used in the room, the absence of pendentive vaults, the sealed wall niches–indicate later construction.

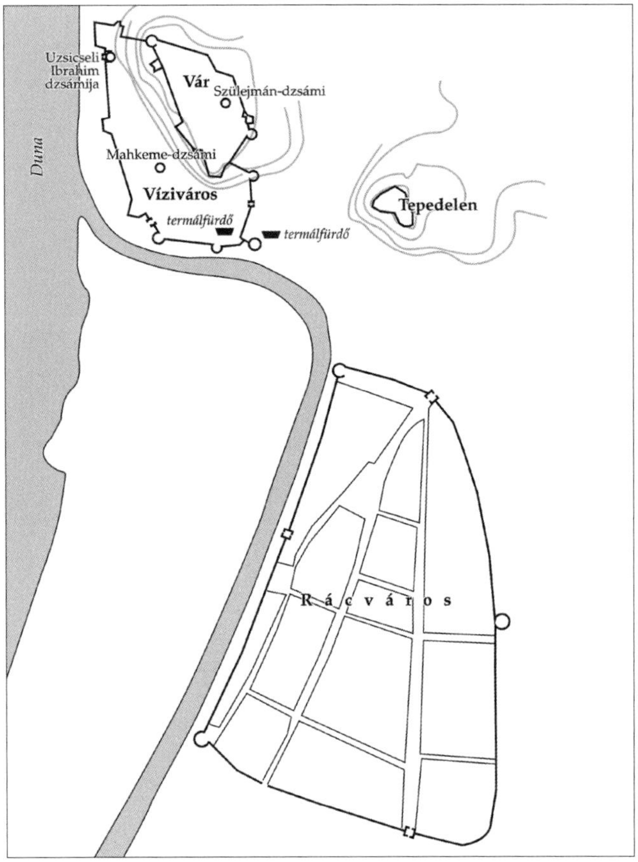

Figure 44. Excavation of the Turkish baths in Esztergom

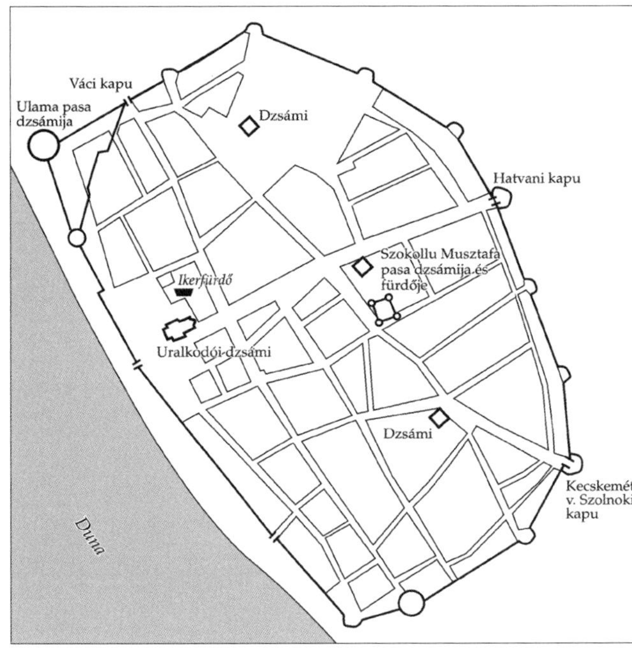

Figure 45. Excavation of the Turkish baths in Pest

In Esztergom, the Grand Vizier Rüstem Pasha and Sokollu Mehmed Pasha had steam baths built, while the thermal waters of the town were utilised in small, 17th-century baths built near one of the bastions of the city wall (*Figure 44*). The hot room of the latter has survived in very good condition, the bottom of its dome and the walls still have the original plaster. The remaining rooms of the baths have not been investigated yet. The baths are clearly discernible in 16th century images, but it is unclear as to which pasha the baths found by the archaeologists belonged.

There were two baths in Pest (*Figure 45*), one of them was discovered by an archaeological excavation at the beginning of the 20th century. The director of the excavation believed it to be an Ottoman structure, but due to a Roman fortress being discovered nearby, the baths were later also declared to be of Roman origin. It was during research begun in 2006, that their Ottoman origin was finally established. The heating and water supply system, the stone material from its furnace room, the layers and infills between the remnants of walls all confirmed this.[43] The ruins of the city's other baths were found during the construction of the University Library. Written sources inform us of their founders: one of them was Güzelje Rüstem Pasha, the other Sokollu Mehmed Pasha.[44]

Two baths are mentioned in 16th century Székesfehérvár, those of Rüstem Pasha and Sokollu Mehmed Pasha.[45] Writing in 1664, Evliya Chelebi only mentions a single double baths,[46] whose ruins were discovered in an excavation in the city centre[47] (*Figure 46*). Images of the other baths survive in etchings produced in 1601,[48] showing a building with a wooden-roofed entrance hall and a dome-covered hot room. These baths stood on the outskirts of the city, next to a mosque.

In addition to the larger Ottoman strongholds listed above, very interesting material has also been found in Babócsa, where, in the area known as the Nárciszos, the baths of the town's commander have been found.

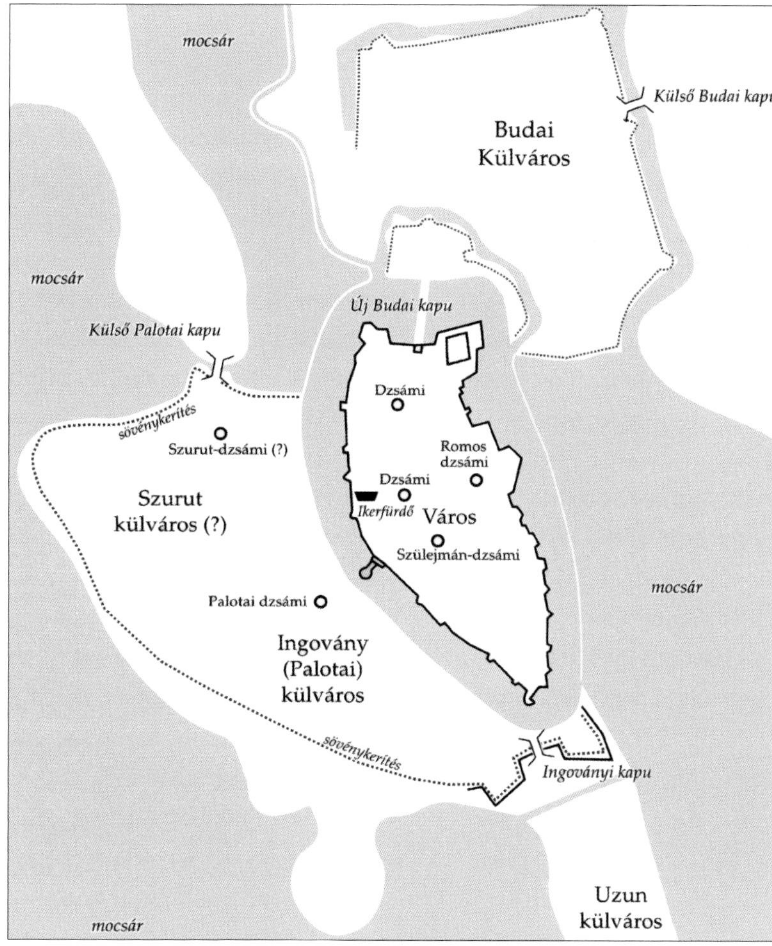

Figure 46. Excavation of the Turkish baths in Székesfehérvár

Reviewing the founding dates of the baths we find that whenever a particular town was conquered, construction projects started within a few years and came to a close within a few decades. The most intense period in that sense were the 1560's and '70's, when Sokollu Mehmed Pasha alone had eight baths built (over ten percent of all the baths built in the occupied territory).[49] With that in mind it is worth considering the number of baths. In cities of the Ottoman Empire of a similar in size to Buda, with populations of eight to ten thousand people, we usually find eight to thirteen baths.[50] Thus Buda's seven built baths and numerous outdoor bathing places were consistent with the imperial average. Similarly, in all other towns, the number of baths sufficient to service the town's population were soon built. The next major changes were brought by the Long War, when, on the one hand, the fighting damaged many buildings, and on the other hand, the steam baths in the towns reconquered by the Hungarians began to deteriorate. When towns were recaptured again by the Ottomans, for instance in Vác, new baths were built, while the 16th-century building was left to crumble.[51]

The social and economic role of Turkish baths

Private initiative played a significant part in the establishment and maintenance of the Ottoman system of social institutions. Mosques, schools, soup kitchens, caravanserais and baths were built, and their founders usually attached them to charitable foundations (*vakf*). These were established for particular purposes, such as the maintenance of a mosque or the operation of a school. In order to be able to achieve their objectives, economic units with revenues–villages, stores, baths, etc.–were attached to the foundation, whose income was then used to perform the tasks defined. These foundations usually remained under the management of the founder's family, thereby also allowing for their assets to be inherited. The baths generated significant revenue, contributing about 10% of the budgets of charitable foundations.[52]

Along with sultans, we also find members of the Ottoman elite among the founders, and they also established baths in the Hungarian occupied territories. Of the forty-six known baths, twenty-three were owned by one of the Buda beylerbeys, six were established by beys, two were maintained by the state, two were founded by the Grand Vizier Rüstem Pasha, while the founders of another thirty baths are unknown. It is clear, therefore, that baths were primarily built by the elite of the occupied territories, while the sites established by the sultan or state formed a small minority. The most prolific commissioners of buildings were naturally the province's most affluent citizens, the Beylerbeys of Buda. Chief among them was Sokollu Mustafa Pasha, who was the head of the Buda *vilayet* for twelve years (1566-1578). He was Bosnian by birth and entered the Sultan's court as payment of child tax. His uncle, Sokollu Mehmed Pasha, had risen all the way to the post of Grand Vizier, and his standing and his power must have played a role in allowing Mustafa Pasha to remain at his post in Buda for so long. After them, the province came to be led by three more members of their family, Ferhad Pasha (1588-1590), Mehmed Pashazade Toygun Pasha, Beylerbey of Buda (1593-1594), who was Grand Vizier Sokollu Mehmed Pasha's son,[53] and Lala Mehmed Pasha (1599-1600, 1601-1602), Grand Vizier Sokollu Mehmed Pasha's cousin. During the period, the Sokollu family was one of the most influential clans of the empire. Kasim Pasha, Beylerbey of Buda (1548-1551, 1557-1558) had baths, a mosque and a monastery built at Pécs, while Buda Pasha Toygun (1553-1556) also had baths built next to his mosque.

Along with the Beylerbeys of Buda, who had high incomes, the beys operating in the province also played their part in the construction projects: Iskender, the Bey of Szigetvár had baths built at Babócsa, while Memi Shah Ghazi and Ferhad Pasha did so in Pécs.[54] All around the occupied territory it was generally the case that people holding office in the province, as well as those with military appointments, conducted some kind of enterprise as well.[55] It was probably for that reason that the Pest judge (*qadi*) and Buda Castle's commander (*dizdar*) both established or owned baths by the natural springs.[56]

Fortunately, a few full foundation inventories survive, in which the founders listed not only the buildings and other economic assets belonging to the foundation, but also attempted to specify their precise locations. Sokollu Mustafa Pasha, for instance, in his inventory of his foundation, wrote as follows: "I hereby attach to my foundation... my caravanserai opposite the Monastery of Hindi Baba, which is near my above-mentioned thermal bath (i.e. the Rudas Baths)."[57] It is also from that data that we have an understanding of the surroundings of baths. Even during that period, the baths aimed to be able to receive the highest possible number of visitors, a certain regularity can be discerned in the sites that were used for those buildings. Some of them were built alongside already operating markets, and those usually had their entrances facing the market. Those that were designed to serve an urban district (*mahalle*) were built in a busy part of the district, next to mosques. And some were part of a complex of buildings (*külliye*), and were built as a single project, using a single design, along with a number of other buildings. Such buildings, which belonged together, were sometimes surrounded by a single shared wall.

Similar factors drove the placement of baths in Hungary, too. Four of the Buda baths were along main roads, with caravanserais and mosques nearby (*Figure 47*). Water from the northern group of thermal springs was utilised by the Császár (Emperor) Baths, which stood by the main road outside the walled city, but there were other buildings nearby: the gunpowder mill, one of Sokollu Mustafa Pasha's mosques, the monasteries of Miftah Baba and Gül Baba, as well as the river port.

Water from the same group of springs was also used by the baths that became today's Király Baths, located along the main road but inside the city walls, near the Cockerel Gate. Sokollu Mustafa's caravanserai and stores operated next door,[58] while the complex containing the pasha's mosque, school and *türbe* were barely 300 metres to the south. At the southern end of the Víziváros district, Toygun Pasha's steam bath was built next to the pasha's mosque. The complex stood by the main road, and there was also a market nearby. Two thermal baths were built to utilise the springs south of the city. The Rudas Baths were also alongside the main road, and as we have already mentioned, it was directly adjacent to Sokollu Mustafa Pasha's caravanserai, while on the other side of the road there was Hindi Baba's monastery, as well as the pasha's mosque and stores.[59] The Rác Baths was built on the edge of a new district, still under construction, but gradually it was surrounded by houses on all sides. It stood by the stream called the Devil's Ditch (Ördög-árok), next to a bridge across the stream, near stores and workshops.[60] In all of the cases described above, there were a number of facilities near the baths building that could supply the required clientele.

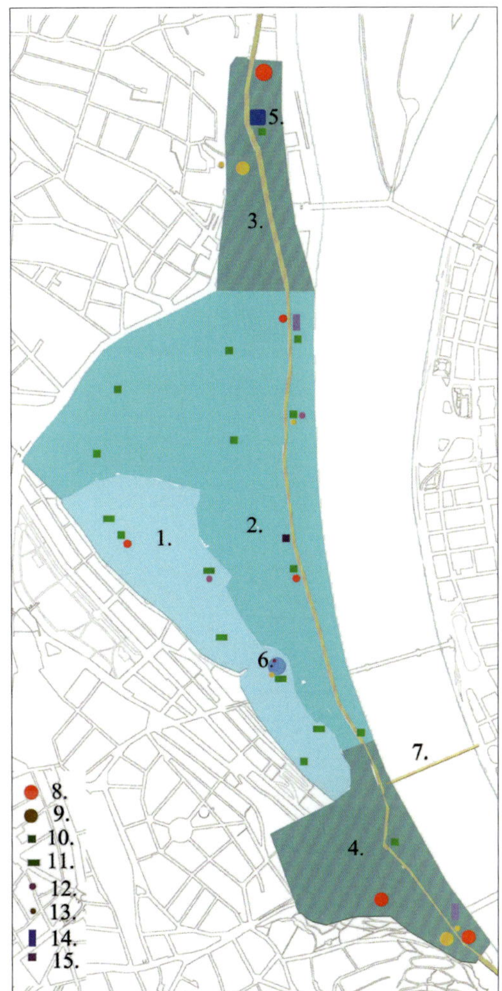

Figure 47. The distribution of Ottoman buildings in Buda. 1. Castle hill. 2. Large suburb. 3. The suburb of Debbaghane. 4. The area of Alhéviz in the Middle Ages. 5. Baruthane. 6. Beylerbey's Palace. 7. Bridge. 8. Bath. 9. Monastery (*tekke*). 10. Newly built mosque. 11. Mosque adapted from a Christian church. 12. Madrasa. 13. Mausoleum. 14. Caravanserai (inn). 15. Warehouse

In the case of both Sokollu Mustafa Pasha and Toygun Pasha, it is clear that they built their baths directly next to other buildings they owned, obviously as a part of an ongoing planning process. The Rác Baths was presumably built to serve the residents of the new district. It was probably highly popular on account of its excellent, very effective medicinal water, as evidenced by the number of extensions that were added to the building.

In Pécs, all three baths stood next to the mosques of the patrons they received their names from (*Figure 48*). The Kasim Pasha Baths were opposite the mosque in the main square, along the city's north-south axis. Along with the mosque, the pilgrimage site of *nisanji* (chancellor) Mehmed Bey was also there, and the city market was also nearby. Memi Pasha's baths also stood alongside the pasha's mosque, and along with his mosque, he also had a madrasa and a drinking fountain there. The complex is located near the Szigetvár Gate. As regards the city's third baths and the mosque next to it, Evliya noted that its community was poor, and that the baths were also for the poor. The two buildings were on two sides of the road connecting the eastern and western city gates, near the monastery also founded by the pasha. Ferhad Pasha's Baths were

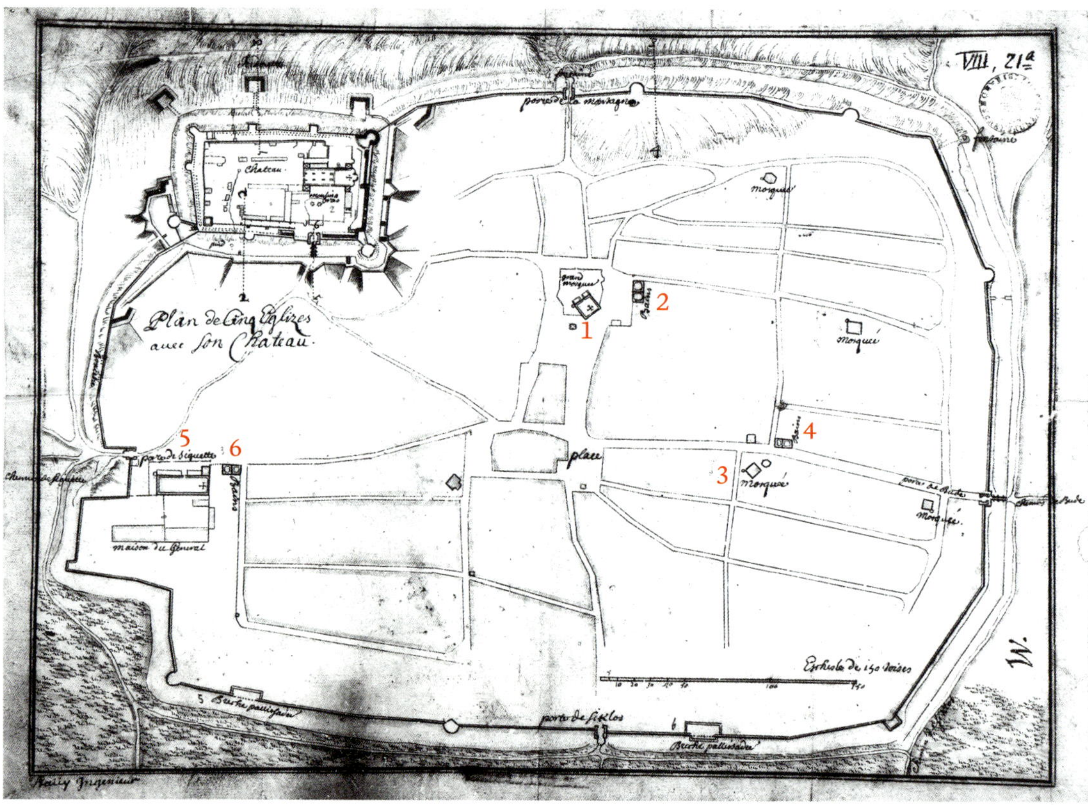

Figure 48. Pécs on Joseph de Haüy's map, 1687. 1. The Kasim Pasha Mosque. 2. The Kasim Pasha Baths. 3. The Ferhad Pasha Mosque. 4. The Ferhad Pasha Baths. 5. The Memi Pasha Mosque. 6. The Memi Pasha Baths

in all likelihood built to serve the district, while Kasim Pasha's Baths were perhaps associated with the expanding city centre. Memi Pasha converted a mediaeval church to a mosque, and also established a number of other things around it. Although he also used existing building, it is still the complex with the strongest sense of a unified plan.

In Pest, Sokollu Mustafa Pasha also established a number of institutions in a single location: his double baths, his caravanserai and his stores are all next to his mosque. The pasha had the mosque built, and although he makes no claims about the baths in the inventory of his foundation, the presence of the caravanserai indicates that a complex may have been built contemporaneously.

The only steam baths in Eger of whose location we are aware was close to the city gate (*Figure 49*). There was also a mosque built nearby[61] and, according to tradition, the plot opposite the baths was the site of an Ottoman school.[62]

We are not aware of any public buildings built other than the baths in Esztergom. Sokollu Mustafa Pasha's foundation inventory generally mentions the nearby buildings as well, but in the case of Esztergom, there are none on the

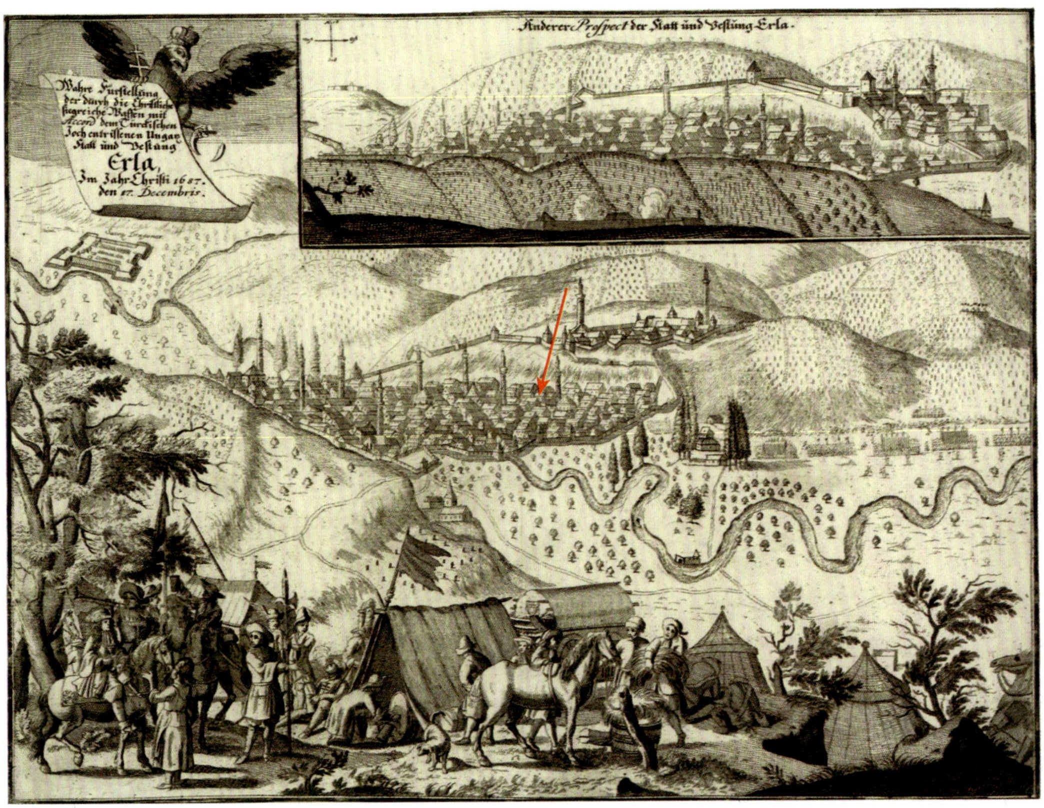

Figure 49. View of Eger, 1687. The red arrow points to the location of the steam baths

list. This indicates that it is highly likely that the pasha himself had none built. Grand Vizier Rüstem Pasha had a mosque built in the city, whose location we are unaware of–it may have stood near his baths.[63]

As in Hungarian territory, the conquerors had to promote their culture, as well as establish the institutions of their religion, the construction of baths was usually related to the building of individual mosques. The founder created a new compound in the city, which had religious buildings (mosques), social functions (soup kitchens, caravanserais) and educational institutions (*mektebs*, madrasas), and it also often included baths. The purpose of such a complex of buildings was to establish them in a central role in the life of the city, so accordingly they were almost always built along the main roads of their respective settlements. We have seen that the majority of the baths were built in the first decades after the conquest, and consequently the buildings of wealthier patrons are often all located in a single *külliye*. Due to the scarcity of information, it is difficult to estimate the extent to which smaller baths and those endowed by the sultan, specifically built to serve individual urban districts, were present in occupied Hungary. In the largest cities (Buda, Pécs), complexes built according to integrated plans dominated. While in the central regions of the Ottoman Empire, among 16th-century buildings, *mahalle*-baths and *külliye*-baths are clearly distinguished,[64] in the newly organised provinces that distinction is not so sharp. In the centres under construction in the occupied territories, the institutions and social facilities required by the conquerors had to be created and organised without local precursors. Those towns had no Muslim populations beforehand, so there were no old Muslim quarters either, where new baths would have had to be built. Consequently, the Ottoman baths were clearly connected to the settling in of the conquerors.

The characteristics of Turkish bath buildings

The structure of Ottoman baths followed a rigid format in the 16th century. One reason for this lay in the water supply system of baths, while on the other hand the characteristic architecture of baths had already become developed fully by the classic era. The strict ground plan conventions were accompanied by a spartan interior: There have been very few discoveries of plastic ornamentation although these had been fairly common in earlier centuries. The ornamentation of baths was provided by minor shifts in plane between architectural elements through which shadows would divide the buildings.

Almost all Turkish baths in Hungary have been destroyed over the centuries. Steam baths can only be surveyed using archaeological methods because, following the wars of reconquest, the new residents did not understand how Ottoman baths were operated, and thus did not use them properly. They were quite evidently unable to use the steam baths as baths. In some cases, these were used to manufacture saltpetre or simply as warehouses and then, as the buildings grew older, they were demolished. Sometimes the side wall of a bathhouse was incorporated into some newer building, preserving the high, aspiring walls of Ottoman buildings, such as in Székesfehérvár (*Figure 50*) or Eger (*Figure 51*). In other cases, however, such as in Pest or Buda, the *hamams* of the 16th and 17th centuries were completely demolished.

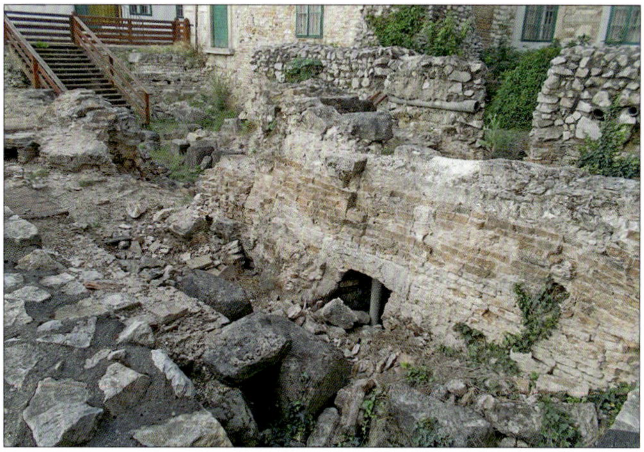

Figure 50. The ruins of the Ottoman era baths in Székesfehérvár

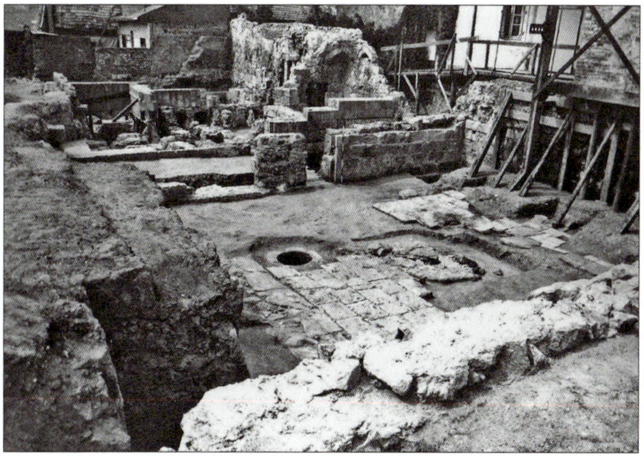

Figure 51. The ruins of the Valide Sultan Baths in Eger

Thermal Baths (*ilijas*) were more fortunate since they had always had pools and their healing properties were widely known, which is why we have been able to find four of them that have been used almost continuously as baths. Nevertheless, the same phenomenon encountered with the steam baths can be noted in these buildings, too. The system of the building was unfamiliar and strange so, following the wars of reconquest, the reconstruction of the baths was consistent with the bathing habits of Christian culture. The fate of the entrance halls shows how these spaces failed to match Hungarian bathing culture in the 18th century: removed from their original context, these buildings may well have seemed like huge halls devoid of any function. Consequently, they were very quickly divided into smaller rooms by partition walls where pools were then constructed. For some reason, the wooden ceilings of the lobbies rapidly disappeared after the reoccupation (they may have been burnt down in the raging fire when Buda was reoccupied). As a result, only the exterior walls and parts of the floors of the remaining thermal baths have been preserved, but absolutely none of their ceiling vaults. By an odd coincidence, these spaces and not the hot rooms covered by cupolas were also bombed in the Second World War. Overall, most of the entrance halls of Ottoman thermal baths were destroyed, while the warm and hot rooms continue to exist more or less in their original Ottoman form with some modification.

Their eastern appearance has meant that the origin of today's functioning Turkish baths in Buda have not been forgotten. The historical research of the buildings was part of the exploration of the history of Buda and Pest in the Ottoman era. In his work entitled *Buda és Pest a török korban* [Buda and Pest in the Ottoman Era], (1944) Lajos Fekete identified the baths and determined the location of the demolished buildings. Evaluations of the buildings in particular were also prepared around this time, following the architectural surveys.[65] The survey of the buildings gathered momentum during the reconstruction following the devastation of the Second World War. Under the leadership of Győző Gerő in most cases, the amount of archaeological research conducted into historical monuments alongside construction varied at that time. There was a new chance to survey these buildings in the early 2000s because by that time the baths had become so worn out and obsolete that their modernisation and renovation required large-scale intervention. Within that framework, surveys of the buildings could be performed, this time using more modern means in which my research fellow was Judit Lászay, the art historian. Only the renovation of The Király Baths remains ahead for us in this century.

The entrance hall

The entrance hall is usually the single largest room of the baths, a capacious square room located on the street front of the building. It can be covered by a cupola or a wooden joisted roof. In the Hungarian cases these have generally been destroyed, leaving only the bases of their walls or survey drawings; from which it seems that wooden joisted roof would have been the most common solution because the walls (based on their thickness) would not have been able to bear the weight of a cupola. The floor structure is known from archaeological data in addition to the standing walls in several cases. The floor was mostly made of large stone paving slabs, and stone was used for the foundation of the bench running along the walls, which was also covered by large stone slabs. The width of the bench varied, but extended to two metres in places. The remains of the niches used for shoes could be identified in both the bath in Pest and the Memi Pasha Baths in Pécs.

Walls were divided by windows and niches. The system of niches was preserved most intact at the Rác Thermal Baths in Buda where six of them were constructed next to one another (*Figure 52*). The starting point of the ceiling vault

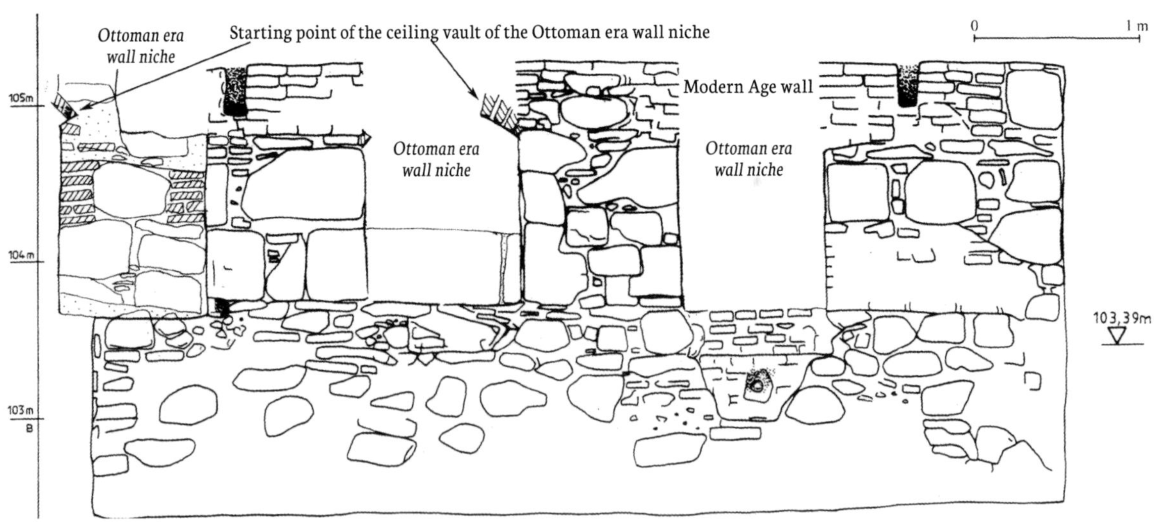

Figure 52. The drawings of the Ottoman era wall niches excavated at the Rác Baths in Budapest, 2009

of the niches and the original plaster on the walls and inside the niches have also survived the ravages of history. The parapets of the niches were explored in the entrance hall of the Valide Sultan Bath in Eger. The walls were covered in pink or red plaster coloured with powdered brick, or sometimes with white plaster. There is insufficient plaster remaining on the walls to reconstruct the changes in colours in the rooms over time. The use of the material itself was not unusual in Ottoman architecture; we can find similar plasters in baths in Turkey.

An ornamental fountain was located in the entrance hall, usually in the centre of the room. The foundations of fountains like this were found in the Memi Pasha Baths in Pécs as well as in the Valide Sultan Bath in Eger. Fragments of a fountain were discovered in Pécs, based on which Győző Gerő was able to prepare a reconstruction of the fountain (*Figure 53*). Nevertheless, they might also have diverted from the established model in the case of the entrance hall, perhaps as a result of some geographic circumstance. The Rác Thermal Baths in Buda are a case in point, the entrance hall there shows interesting, unique solutions from several perspectives. It is not a regular square in shape because the building had to be squeezed in between Gellért hill and a stream. Its direction and shape was determined by a fissure in the rock of the spring supplying the bath with water which, was included into the entrance hall. These factors caused several differences from the common floor plan: the organisation of the rooms of the bath, the location of the entrance and the bench above the catchment are all different from usual. Even the fountain is not found in the middle of the hall: it is unique in Hungary that it was built sunk into the steps of the bench. (*Figure 54*)

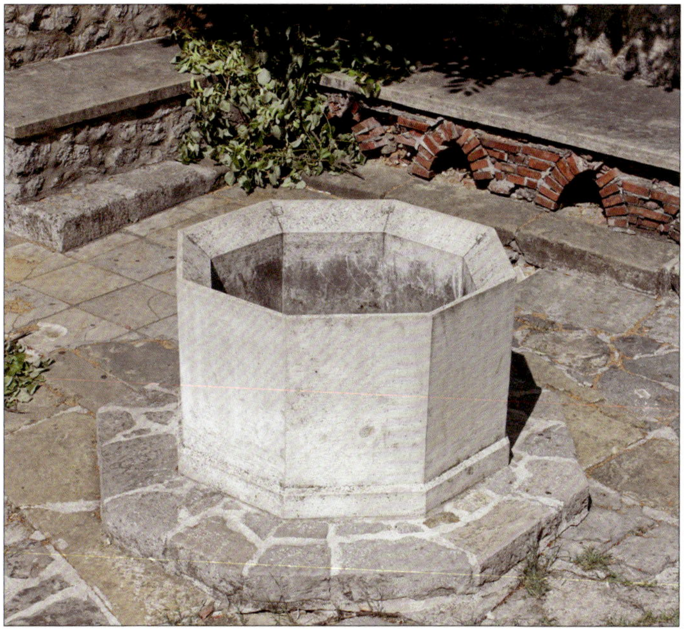

Figure 53. The well excavated and reconstructed in the entrance hall of the Memi Pasha Baths

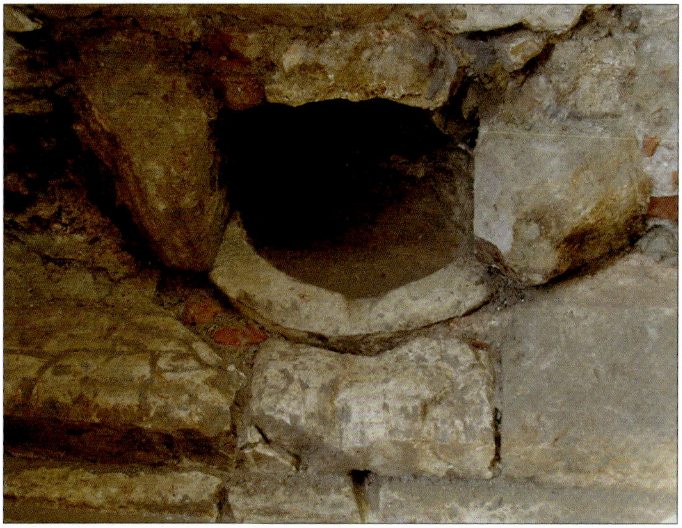

Figure 54. A well sunk beneath a stairway in the excavated entrance hall of the Rác Baths, photographed from above

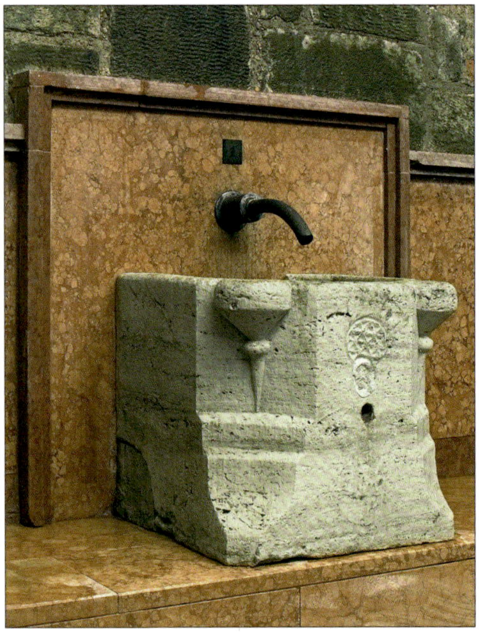

Figure 55. An original stone basin (*kurna*) at the Rudas Baths

The warm rooms

The following sequence of rooms consists of warm rooms, which filled the rectangular space between the two square spaces of the entrance hall and the hot room in the baths in Hungary, typically in 16th-century buildings. In smaller baths, for example in the Memi Pasha Baths in Pécs, the Rác Thermal Baths in Buda or in the double bath in Székesfehérvár, this is one single room while in larger buildings–for example in the Rudas and Császár Baths–they are divided into a number of parts. These spaces are usually covered by brick annular vaults, but at the Császár baths, for example, a trough vault can be found. Skylights–small windows in the vault ceilings–were placed in the vault ceilings through which the accumulating steam could also escape. An interesting solution in the Rác Thermal Baths was a window, opened on one of the shorter sides, and accordingly skylights used only in the places farther away from the window.

The warm rooms were wet spaces where wall fountains were situated on the stone bench along the walls. The floor heating system also reached across them in the steam baths. The pool of wall fountains (*kurna*) were constructed of approx. 40 cm stone cubes the inside of which were carved into a basin the edges of which were often decorated. These stone basins did not have drains; the water flowed on the floor (*Figure 55*). A tap or taps were installed in the small stone slab above the basins from which the water could be drained.

Niches were cut into the walls in which to place the tools used for bathing. In the warm room of the Rác Thermal Baths a small pool was constructed during a conversion, most probably due to the huge number of guests at the baths which were famous for their healing properties.

The toilet

The toilet was most often placed in the centre of the baths, often opening from the warm room. The waters from the floor of the bath were led towards the walled and stone-covered toilet, and sewage was drained off the building through the channel built underneath. This channel is very well preserved in the Rác Thermal Baths where it is in the same block as the building. The foundation of this was thought to have been exposed at the Rudas Baths where, however, it was outside the uniform block of the building. The same can be observed in the case of the Valide Sultan Baths in Eger.

The hot room

The hot room is the innermost and hottest room of the baths. Most of the information we have is about this part because in the still operating thermal baths from the Ottoman era these rooms have been preserved in their most intact state. The hot room was covered by a brick-laid cupola in every case (*Figure 56*). Two methods were used to vent the accumulating steam and to let light in: either the cupola was broken by small skylights, mostly placed in concentric circles, or a single, large, circular opening (*opeion*) was placed in the centre of the cupola with a small tower-like structure outside (*Figure 57*). Skylights were constructed in the Császár, Rudas and Király Baths, while we presume there was an opeion at the Rác Thermal Baths.

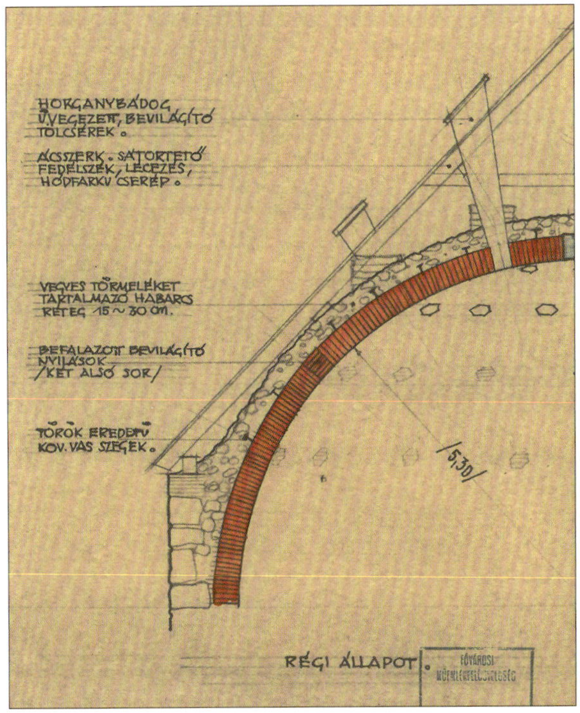

Figure 56. Survey made from the roof of the Király Baths in Buda, 1962

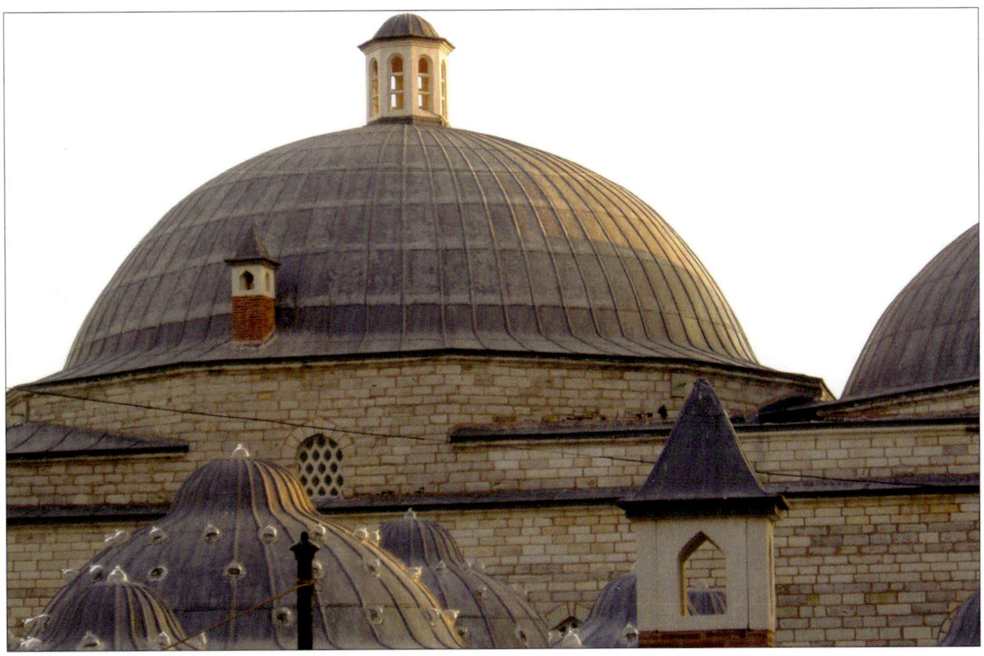

Figure 57. The *opeion* that can be seen at the Bajezid II Baths in Istanbul, late 15th – early 16th century

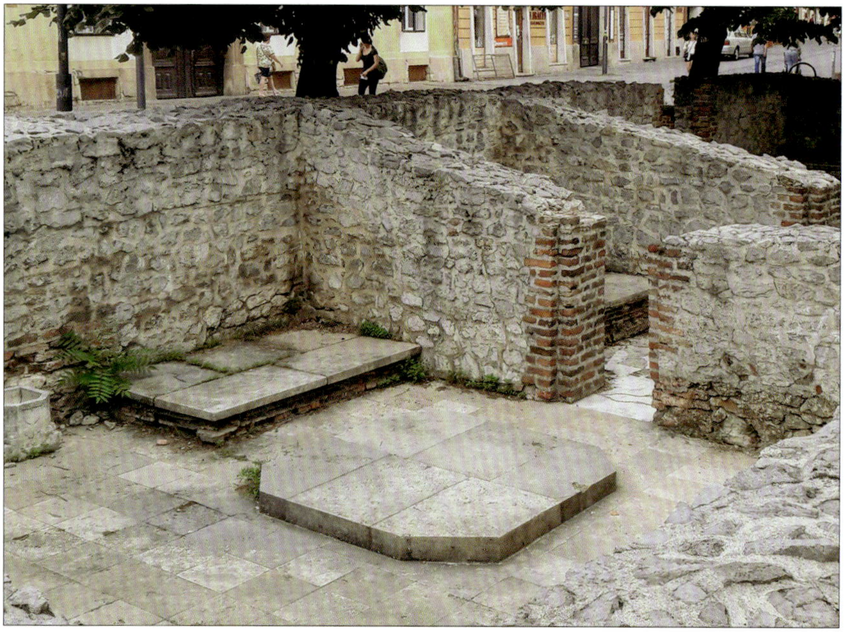

Figure 58. The reconstructed naval stone at the Memi Pasha Baths

Plastered walls are found along the stone-covered floor and benches. Pink or red lime plaster coloured with brick dust or white lime plaster was used here as well. A sufficiently large area of plaster from the 16th and 17th centuries was preserved at the Császár Baths for the system of these three colours actually to be studied (for more detail see the chapter discussing ornamentation).

Wall fountains were placed beside the walls, the external surface of which was plastered in the same colour as the wall. This solution was easily observed in the Rác Thermal Baths where the impressions of the pools of the wall fountains were preserved on the floor, as well as the plaster facing them on the wall. The impression of the stool upon which elderly or ill people could sit was also preserved on the floor.

At the centre of the hot rooms at the steam baths stood the so called naval stone; a raised platform constructed from and covered in stone (*Figure 58*). A small part of this came to the surface in the double bath in Pest; however, only the floor heating system constructed beneath it refers to its former presence at other steam baths. The naval stone was most frequently octagonal in shape, and the organisation of the columns of the floor heating system also follows this form. This is how we know that the naval stones of Valide Sultan Baths in Eger and the Memi Pasha Baths in Pécs were also octagonal.

The centre of the hot room of the Thermal Baths was occupied by the pool which is octagonal and four steps deep in each of the Hungarian examples. The steps, made of large stone blocks, run around the entire pool. The top step was raised slightly above the floor around it, preventing the flow of dirty water from the floor into the pool (*Figure 59*).

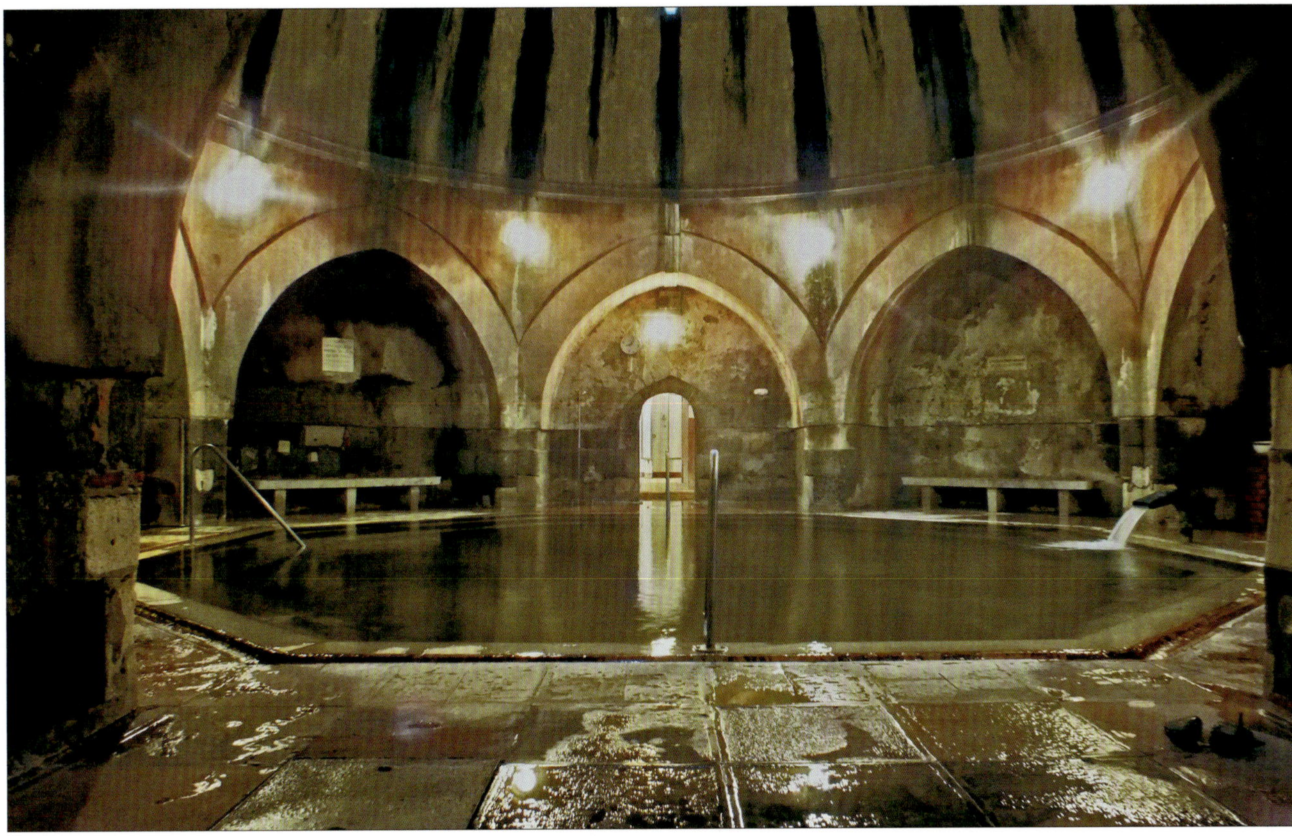

Figure 59. The hot room at the Király Baths

The re-cycling of stone from old buildings from the neighbourhood was a common practice in Ottoman construction works, sometimes even from other towns. That is why two renaissance carvings from the Royal Castle of Buda are to be found among the floor stones at the Rác Thermal Baths in Buda (*Figure 60*). We know from written sources that stones were shipped from great distances like Pécs for the construction works of Toygun Pasha.[66]

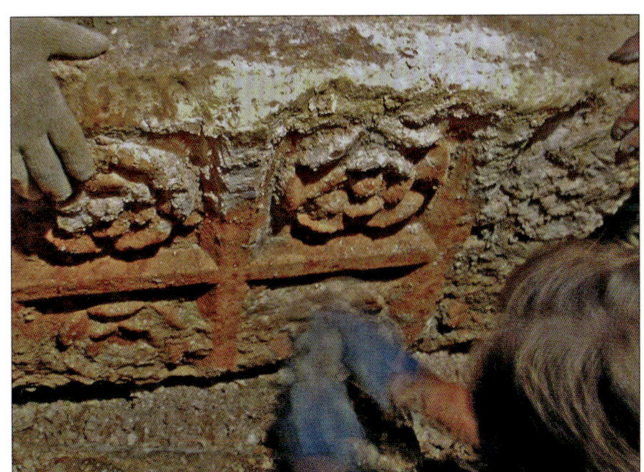

Figure 60. A piece of renaissance red marble emerging from the floor of the hot room at the Rác Baths during excavation

Private baths

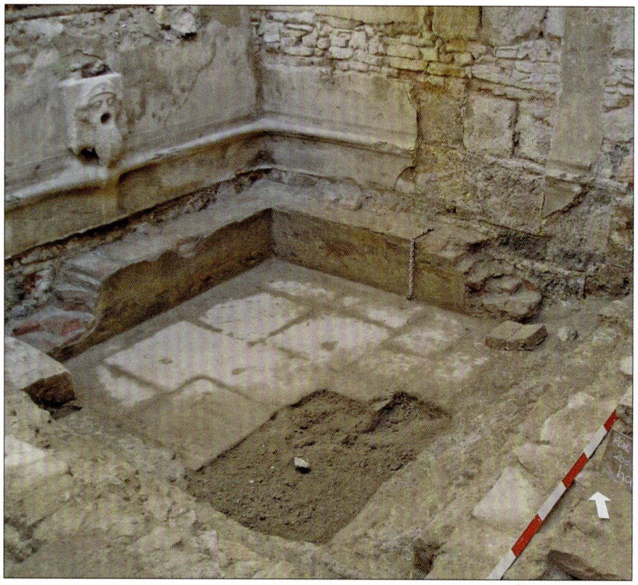

Figure 61. The private bath at the Rác Baths during excavation

Smaller square-shaped rooms were connected to the hot room of most baths. Such private baths were certainly not constructed at the Rudas Baths, although a wooden structure dividing the space could be imagined within the large cupola space. In the cases of other Hungarian baths, these rooms can be clearly identified where stone benches were often built along the walls and wall fountains were placed on these. We know two private baths in which such pools were built: one is the Rác Thermal Baths and the other the Császár Baths. These pools are square-shaped, following the shape of the room, and they are similar in style to the pool of the hot room. In the case of the Rác Thermal Baths it was fitted into one of the corners and steps were built on its other two sides. A layer of plaster can be found on the side walls of the room that runs down to the floor of the pool (*Figure 61*).

Water treatment system

The operation of baths requires significant technical infrastructure, so heating, and draining water and the sewage system were an important part of the construction of the buildings.[67] The water treatment system of thermal and steam baths is significantly different. The only similarity found is that water is lead from the cisterns to the wall fountains (and the pools) through ceramic water pipes in the walls (*Figure 62*). The pipes frequently required replacement, so sometimes white glazed or red, sometimes unglazed pipes were excavated alongside each other. A larger space was left for the pipes in the walls and the area of the pipes was built from brick so they could ensure the necessary slope more easily. Water was led by gravitation, i.e. by the slope of the pipes from the tanks, which were built higher than to the fountains. In the Rudas Baths in Buda we could also see that textile had been wound around the pipes at the joints for sealing, the lime scale impression of which is preserved on the water pipes placed in the wall of the warm room. There are also traces in the same bath indicating that a separate pipeline system was installed in the wall to fill the pool that had larger diameter pipes that only led to the pool. The pipelines filling the other pools have degenerated so much that we can no longer form a clear picture of them. The water flowing over the floor was drained by surface channels towards the toilet where it was drained into the sewage channel.

The water was led from the constructed tanks to the pipes running in the walls. There is a significant difference between thermal and steam baths in the location of the tanks. The cisterns in the steam baths had precisely determined locations: behind the hot rooms, extending to their entire width. Only the heating house was further back. The tank was around the size of a huge room. A fire burned beneath its floor and the round opening of the fireplace was covered with copper above which was placed the water (see *Figure 30*). The air heated up by the fire was led partly under the tank and partly under the building, i.e. the hot and the warm rooms. The floor of the hot and the warm rooms was supported by short brick columns (*Figure 63*) around which hot air flowed before being let out of the building through the vertical pipes built into the walls. These short brick columns were found by Győző Gerő in the case of the Memi Pasha Baths in Pécs, the Valide Sultan Baths in Eger and the double baths in Székesfehérvár. Fortunately, in the case of the double bath in Pest the floor was also preserved and the small columns of the *hypocaustum* (the under-floor heating system) underneath are also intact. A cold-water tank was also placed next to the hot water tank. The walls of both were used as access to the wall fountains through the abovementioned water pipelines. As a result, two water pipes were always led under each other in steam baths, and we can find two taps at the wall fountains too, one for cold and one for hot water.

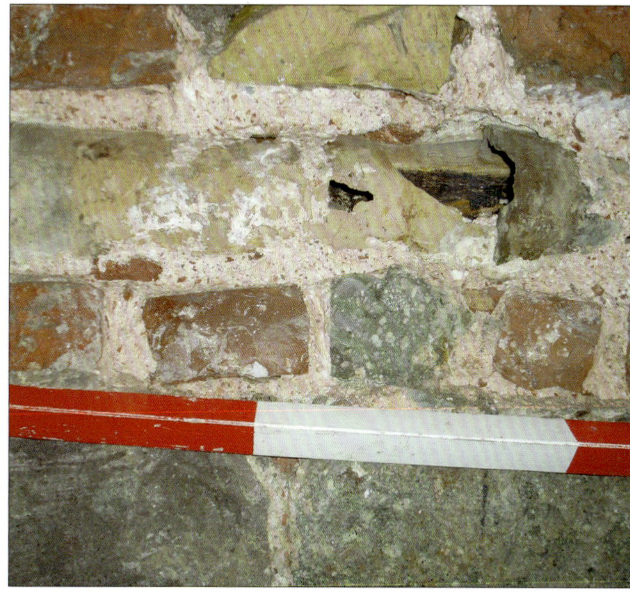

Figure 62. Ottoman era ceramic waterpipes excavated from the wall at the Rudas Baths

Since they didn't have to heat water in thermal baths, the heating house was unnecessary. The location of the tank was determined by the thermal spring. The tank itself had a dual function: on the one hand to catch and store the water; and on the other to raise the water level in order for gravity to send it down to the baths. Consequently, several interconnected tanks could be made around the bath. The spring breaks through to the surface from a 12-metre fissure in the rock at the Rác Thermal Baths that lies below the entrance hall of the building. The edge of the rock was raised, and a tank was built around it. The floor level of the stone bench was built far higher than usual above the spring, so they could elevate the level of water above the height of the water pipelines of the interior rooms. In the Császár Baths they used another interesting solution. On the one hand they used both a cold and a hot water spring, so as opposed to the other Thermal Baths in Buda where there are two water pipelines running in the walls. We do not know the springs that were used. All we know is that there is a well next to the southern side of the bath the surroundings of which were formed in the Ottoman era. Its water was channelled away, possibly unused. At the same location two small tanks were built next to the wall of the bath from outside in which water pipelines run, however we do not know the starting point of these. There is no floor heating under the floor of the thermal baths because the buildings were heated by the large amount of thermal water.

The fountains in the lobbies were supplied with water by a small separate tank. This had to be placed high in the vicinity of the entrance hall in order to ensure sufficient water pressure. The water pipe supplying the well was preserved at the Valide Sultan Baths in Eger where it was led from one corner of the room to the well under the floor.

The water used in the baths had to be drained from the building. Relatively little water was used in steam baths and it left the building in two channels: one drained the water of the fountains from the entrance hall by the shortest route; while the other, a stone-walled channel, left the building at the toilet taking sewage out with it. Similar channels were also built in the thermal baths, but the water of each pool was taken out of the building via separate gutters. The water slowly flowing on the floor of the hot room was led to the channel emptying the pool in the Rác Thermal Baths, and the water flowing on the floor of the warm room and the entrance hall was led towards the toilet. At the Rudas Baths the surface channels also sloped towards the toilet and the water from the floor was also led that way.

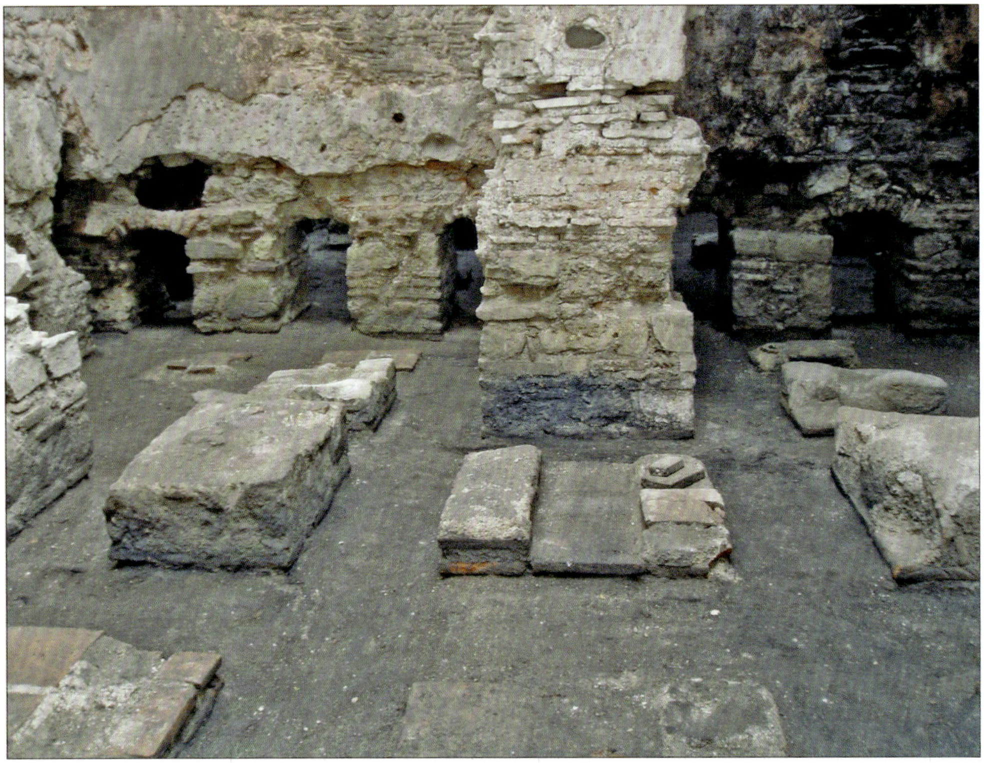

Figure 63. 14th-century columns excavated at the Murad I Baths in Iznik that were part of the underfloor heating system

Ornaments

Ornaments can be best examined in the still existing thermal baths in Buda. Many valuable details were preserved in the Valide Sultan Baths in Eger and the double bath in Székesfehérvár where some of the wall remains standing as far as the beginning of the ceiling vault.

The baths of the 16th century were characterised by sparse ornamentation. The stalactite ornaments widely used in Ottoman architecture are only present on small surfaces. There are delicate hanging stalactite ornaments made of stone in the corners of the hot room in the Rudas Baths (*Figure 64–65*). The version used in the ceiling vaults of the Császár Baths is much simpler and formed simply from cubes (*Figure 66*). Nevertheless, the interesting thing at the Császár Baths is that they prepared ornaments emerging from and recessing into the plane surface, mostly from bricks. In the spaces where the private baths opened out stalactites can be seen emerging from the plane while there are others recessed into the surface in other rooms. Pendulous ornaments were only made on the heads of the pillars of the hot room which are similar to the elements seen at the Rudas Baths. A simple stalactite ornament of brick slightly differing from the one at the Császár Baths can be seen at the baths in Székesfehérvár.

Plastic ornaments were also used at doorways, for example the ogival arch was closed by a stepped ornament (*Figure 67*). Such solutions were uncovered during the exploration of the Rudas, Rác and Császár Baths in Buda. The stepped ornaments above the doors leading to the private baths were combined with stalactites at the Császár Baths.

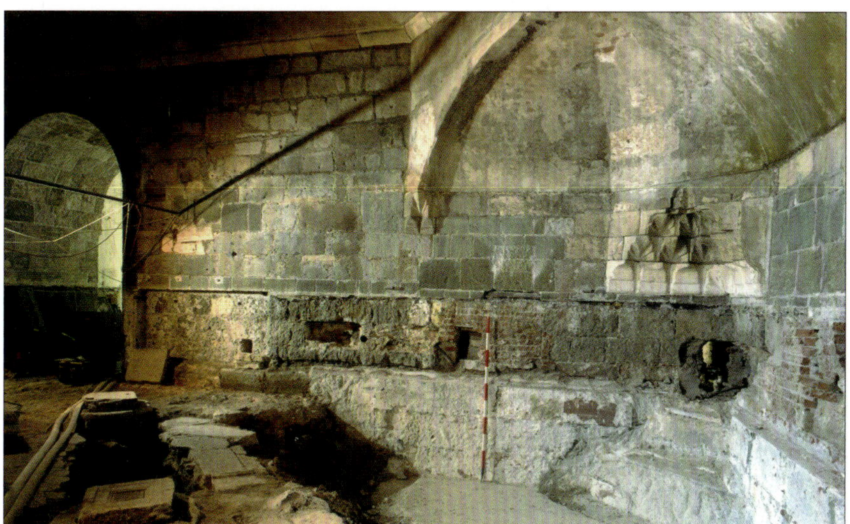

Figure 64. Stalactite decorations visible in the corners of the hot room at the Rudas Baths during excavations

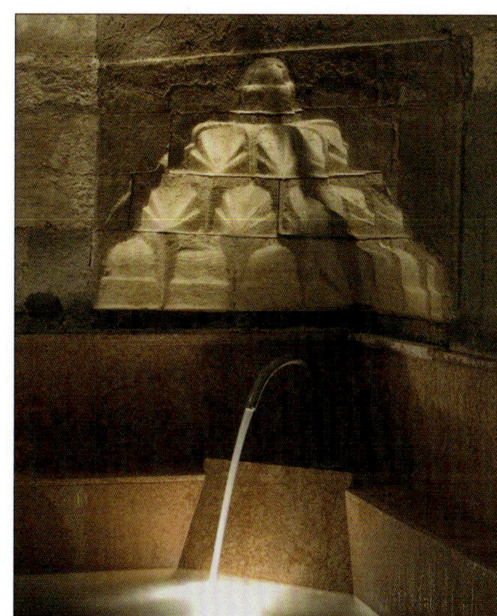

Figure 65. Stalactite decorations visible in the corners of the hot room at the Rudas Baths following restoration

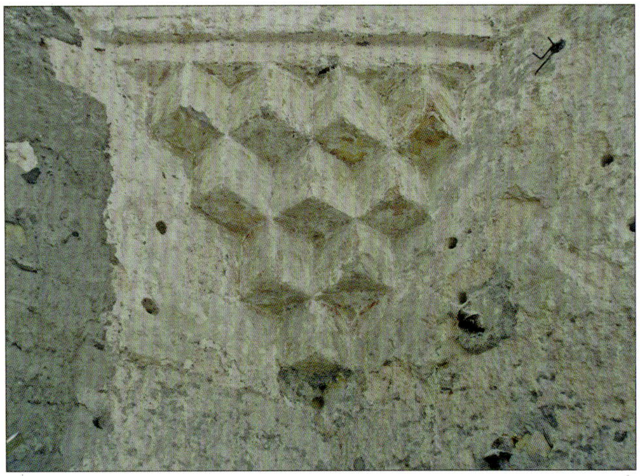

Figure 66. Stalactite decoration in the hot room at the Császár Baths

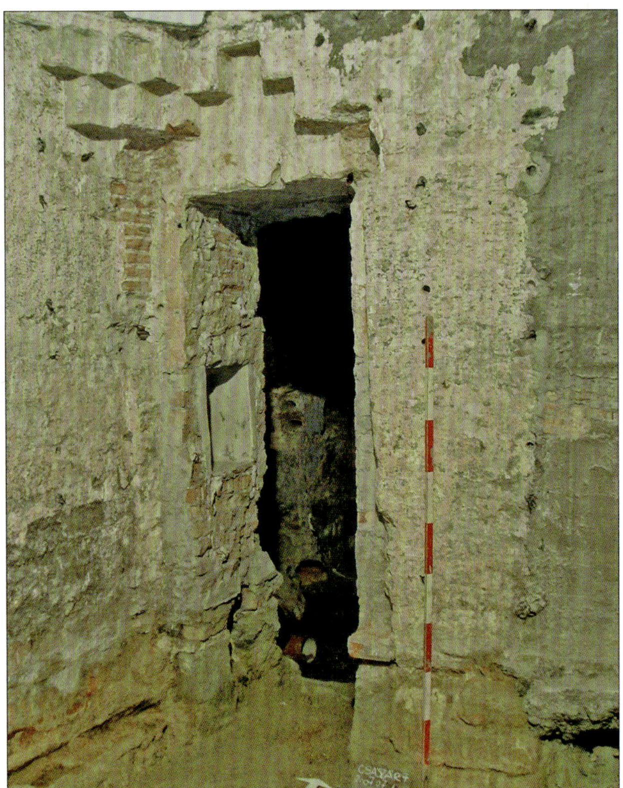

This was, however, only possible on one side of the doorways, and in the cases of doors recessed into the plane of the wall. On the other side, only the ogival arch can be seen today. In the Ottoman era, however, this side of the doors was also more highly ornamented. It was observed at the Császár Baths that the ogival arch was followed by a levelled plaster surface on this side which emphasised the arch of the door. It is assumed that this was prepared in other buildings too, but no sign remains today.

Breaks in the plane of a few centimetres formed at the connections of architectural elements to make the shadows more emphatic and thus decorate the buildings. These ornaments were applied at the beginning of cupolas, along the arch of spandrels, and at the ogee arch closures of large niches.

The colour of plastered walls was not monotonous either. The colour of popular red marble was mimicked, and they polished the plaster hard enough to make it almost water repellent. The size of the plastered surface preserved in Császár Baths was sufficient to prepare colour reconstructions. On the one hand the pink plaster was base plaster on which different coloured plasters or perhaps paint could be applied, and on the other hand this covered ceiling vaults. The side walls were red. In one period at the Császár Baths the bottom of the side walls was coloured red and the walls and the ceiling vaults above were white. Research workers found something interesting in the small bath in Esztergom: they explored an image of a ship carved in the plaster that could have been graffiti rather than the result of conscious decorative purpose. The exterior walls of the buildings were also plastered. Smaller pieces of plaster were explored on the facade of the Császár and Rác Thermal Baths.

Figure 67. Stepped decoration around the doorway to the hot room at the Császár Baths

Niches had an important role in the baths and appeared in groups of three. On the northwestern side of the warm room of the Rác Thermal Baths there is one niche on each side of the door leading to the hot room. Also on the north-western side in the hot room there were originally three niches, but one of them was later converted into a door. These niches are decorative parts of the different rooms.

Lighting

Skylights in the ceiling vaults and windows served the lighting of baths (*Figure 68*). In Hungary, openings on the ceiling vaults can be seen at the Thermal Baths in Buda. Generally hexagonal skylights are found in these buildings, with the exception of the Császár Baths, where they are round. These openings were covered by bell-shaped glass,[68] of which,

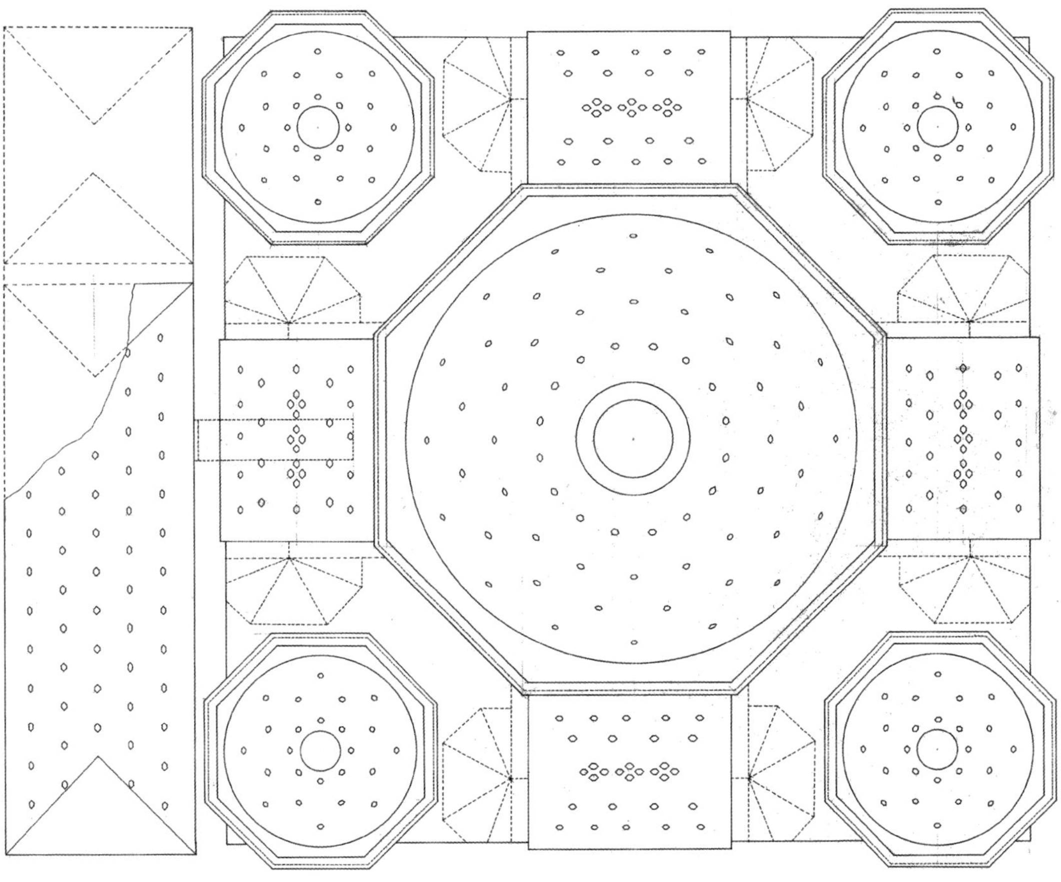

Figure 68. Survey drawings of the vaulting at the Császár Baths, 1974

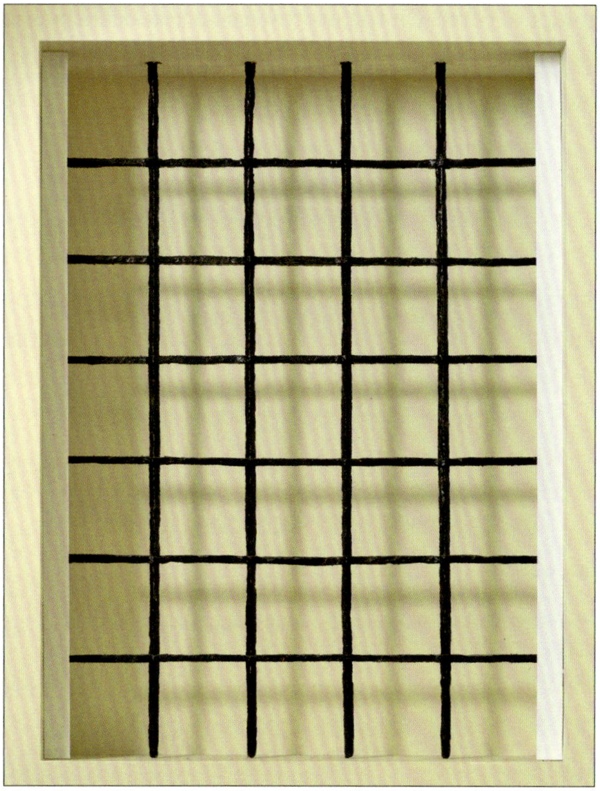

Figure 69. Restored window bars excavated from beside the Rác Baths

however, no archaeological trace is left today. We have no information on the upper structure of the skylight of the ceiling vault (*opeion*) of the hot room in the Rác Thermal Baths. There are no small skylights on the cupola here but there is a large walled up opening in the middle of the cupola. That the architect Miklós Ybl created this is clear from his reconstruction plans prepared in 1890. He began to deal with the reconstruction and extension of the building in the 1860s. Győző Gerő, however, had it walled up during the reconstructions in the 1960s because he didn't think it was related to the Ottoman era. However, the steam had somehow to leave the cupola so there must have been a smaller opening in the middle of it, all signs of which however disappeared during the reconstructions at the end of the 19th century.

In addition to the openings in the ceiling vaults, the buildings were divided by windows too which could appear in any of the rooms if the surroundings of the building allowed it. In the Rác Thermal Bath, where there was a ditch along the side looking to the hill next to the hot and the warm rooms, they could easily open windows because nobody could look in. In contrast, there was surely no window in the warm room of the Rudas Baths, perhaps due to its proximity to the main road. There were windows on the hot room and the private baths of the Császár Baths too. The windows were glazed, evident from the lead frames and glass fragments found in the ditch of the Rác Thermal Baths, mentioned above. A disguarded window rail was also found here (*Figure 69*).

However, the baths were used not only in daylight, but also in the evenings, at which time of day they were lit with oil lamps and candles[69] placed in niches in the walls.[70] No clearly identifiable remains of these have been found in Hungary.

The variety of floor plans

Finally, I shall examine the floor plan solutions of the hot rooms at baths in Hungary. The eight classification groups for Ottoman bath buildings based on the floor plans of their hot rooms have been discussed above (see *Figure 33*). Taking the hundreds of baths around the Ottoman Empire into consideration, the most popular floor plan solution

is evidently the cross-shaped baths (A), followed by the central cupola (E), the uniform size cupola (F), the star-shaped (B), the square-shaped (C), the multiple cupola (D), the single cupola (H) and finally the column hot room (G). The most common floor plan type is the cross, and far fewer baths fall into the other categories, with hardly any buildings in the column group. In contrast to this, in Hungary the various types of floor plans are represented in almost equal numbers among the baths. In order of frequency: the single cupola (H), the star-shaped (B), the central cupola (E), the cross-shaped (A), and the column (G). There are no examples of the square (C), the multiple cupola (D) or the uniform sized cupola (F) types.

Despite the small number of baths explored in Hungary, unique solutions can also be found. The Császár Baths represent the cross groundplan type, the most popular type around the empire, but one with many unusual details. Most notable is the size of the building, which is much larger than most Ottoman baths. Furthermore, the individual baths do not open from the central cupola space. The *iwans* are organised in an interesting way because, rather than simply having four large *iwans* opening from the cupola space, there are actually twice that number, with the spaces at the sides arranged as if two *iwans* had been turned to face each other. We do not know any other baths in the territory of the Ottoman Empire built with precisely this design feature. The Rudas Bath is also unique and amazes the visitor at first sight by its huge size. The cupola resting on columns is such a rare floor plan solution that there are barely any other examples anywhere across the empire. The two baths in Istanbul comparable to the Rudas in terms of floor plan—Sultan Süleyman the Magnificents' steam bath and Sokollu Mehmed Pasha's baths in Azapkapı—are the works of Mimar Sinan. Grand Vizier Sokollu Mehmed Pasha was Sokollu Mustafa's uncle, so it may not be a coincidence that the two baths had the same name: *Yeshil Direkli Hamam* (bath with green columns).

Examples comparable to the double baths in Pest can also be found in Istanbul. It is not the floor plan solution of the hot room that is unusual here, rather the position of the two parts of the bath. The parts of the double baths for men and women were usually placed alongside each other so that the rooms with the same function would connect, giving the building as a whole an almost square floor plan. In contrast to this, the two parts of the building of the baths in Pest are connected at the hot rooms, and the lobbies are placed at opposite ends of the building creating a long rectangle. This can be seen in the case of the *Haseki Hürrem Hamami* (steam bath).

The hot room in one half of the double bath in Székesfehérvár shows a combination of two floor plan types. The star-shaped (B) floor plan type was not an octagonal arrangement, but rather a hexagon in which the two private baths were attached in a manner characteristic of the central cupola 'E' type. The reason for this solution was most certainly the small size because three private baths were usually attached to the hexagonal hot room in larger buildings.[71]

The floor plan of the Memi Pasha Baths demanded further consideration. One half of the double bath was explored, in this example, where the base of the building was exposed from the entrance hall to the cistern. The floor had been destroyed in both the warm and the hot rooms, but the columns of the floor heating system were in good condition when they were excavated and referenced the structures above the floor. There are always columns below the naval stone that outline its shape, placed close to each other so that they can support the weight of the platform's structure. Although a pillar solution is also used under the walls between the rooms, it is different from that supporting the floor

because of its function. In the hot room of the Memi Pasha Baths it can be seen that the columns indicating the place of the naval stone are not located in the middle, but closer to the warm room, and the square of the hot room is divided by a wall. Consequently, a floor plan of the central cupola (E) type can be assumed in contrast to the current reconstruction of the historical building.

The incidence of double baths is roughly equivalent to that generally in the Ottoman Empire, i.e. one third of the baths explored in Hungary belong to this group. The floorplans of the Memi Pasha Baths, the Ferhad Pasha Baths and the double bath in Székesfehérvár are known enough to be able to identify the parts for men and women. Only the excavated part of the Memi Pasha Baths could open from the main street so this was the section for men. The street also provided orientation in the case of the Ferhad Pasha Baths. In the early decades of the 20th century, archaeologist and art historian Ottó Szőnyi[72] tried to determine which part of it could have been for women and which part for men. On the drawing by Joseph de Haüy it can be seen that the road in front of the lobbies of the bath led to the gate. The baths were built on a corner and a side street ran along the Western part of the building, thus it may have had an entrance from there. Furthermore, the 18th-century survey drawing shows that the Eastern part of the building is slightly larger than the other side. Based on this, it is possible to conject that the western part might have been the wing for women and the eastern wing for men. Ottó Szőnyi took the opposite view because the floor plan of the western part is more complex than the other side. Nevertheless, the lesson to be learnt in studying double baths in Turkey is that it is essentially the size and the position that counts, while the floor plan type is less important in identifying the parts for men and women in double baths.

The place of baths in Hungary within Ottoman architecture

In the following, an answer is sought to the questions of how standard the bath buildings in the occupied territory are, whether they have any local characteristics, and with what regions they have demonstrable connections. We have seen that the number of baths in Buda (seven) conforms with the tendency seen in the Ottoman Empire, as well as the two or three baths of smaller towns. Two baths in Buda, the Rudas and the Császár, are outstanding among the bath buildings in Hungary due to their size. Originally, they may have been approximately 20 by 45 metres. Such gigantic baths were rare in the Ottoman Empire, only the really big ones like the double Baths of Sultan Bayezid in Istanbul (34 by 48 metres) or Yeni Kaplija (New Baths, 31 by 47 metres) in Bursa can be compared to the large thermal baths in Buda in terms of size. The smaller baths in Buda were around 15 by 35 metres while the Ferhad Pasha Baths in Pécs are around 26 by 21 metres. Considering the above, most bath buildings in Hungary are average in size and the two baths in Buda are very large (*Figure 70*).

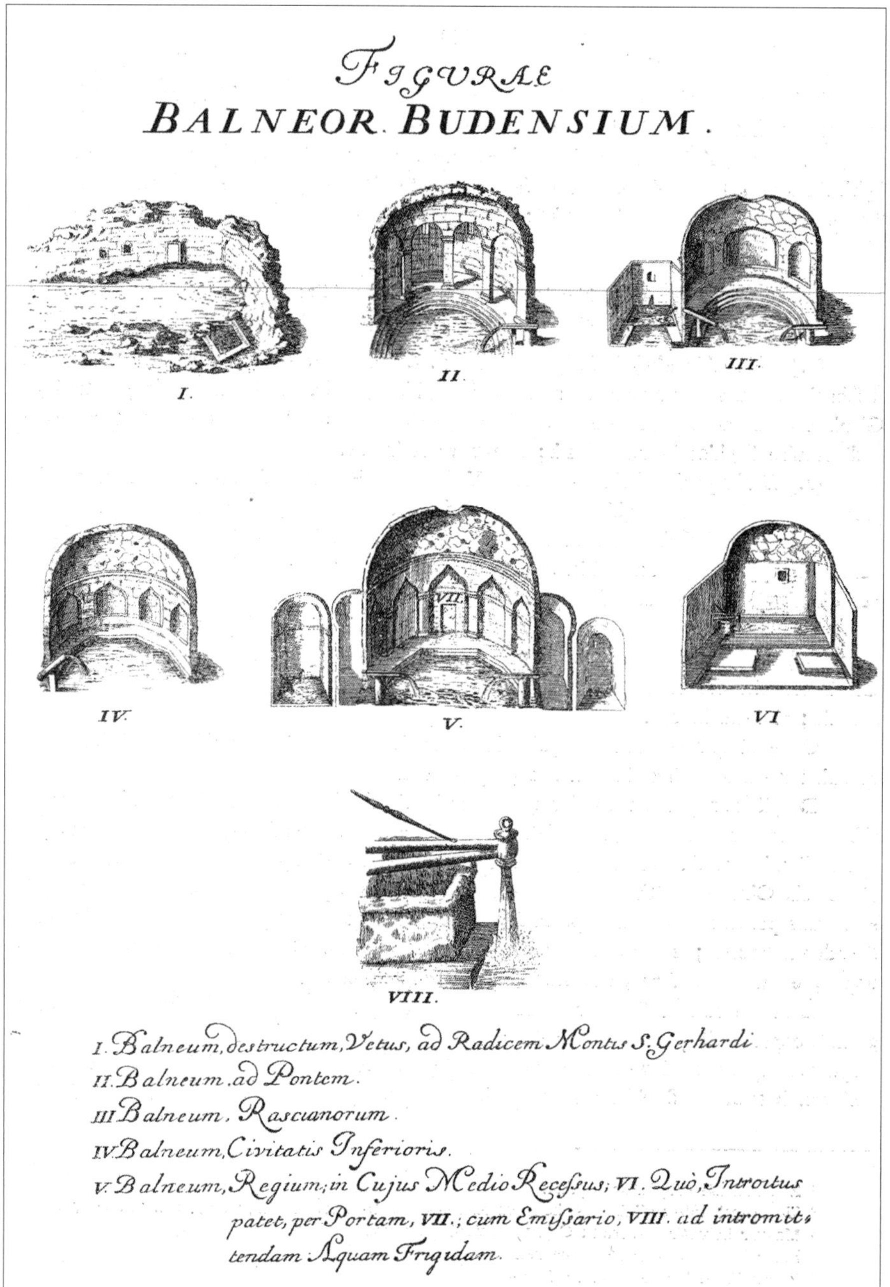

Figure 70. Schematic drawings of the baths of Buda from the Luigi Ferdinando Marsigli collection, late 17th century

Among Ottoman bath buildings many double bath buildings can be found, one third of all baths fall into this category. However, among thermal baths in the Ottoman Empire–most of the baths in Buda fall into this category–this building type is definitely atypical. Only two of the eleven known thermal baths in Bursa are double baths. The reason for this may be the large amount of water required and the complex water supply system. Consequently, the situation in Buda fits the standard across the Empire well: on the one hand the thermal baths are all single in form and on the other hand one of the two public steam baths in the city was a double bath. In other towns we do not know in each case whether the given bath was a double bath or not, so the incidence of double baths cannot be examined in the whole of Ottoman Hungary. It is certain that there are several double baths among the explored baths, so their incidence cannot not be ignored.

The Császár Baths and the steam bath in Eger belong to the most common type of baths with four *iwans*, that is, private baths on each of the corners. The bath in Eger[73] shows the general characteristics of this type while the Császár Baths are outstanding with their unique solutions. The Császár Baths differ from comparable baths in three ways: on the one hand the rectangular space of the iwans opening from the hot room includes two additional iwans. On the other hand, the private baths in the corners do not open from the central part of the hot room, rather from the iwans. This structure is similar to the star floor plan, providing an opportunity to place large niches around the pool in the centre. Most interestingly, these two elements very rarely appear as such. The two floor plan solutions of the building show old elements that were more common in the 15th century: such is the rectangular shape of the space between the private baths and the placement of the entrances to the private baths opening from the spaces on the sides. The further structure and decoration of the iwans is characteristic of the Császár Baths, which follow a really rare design (*Figure 71*). Based on this we can say that the organisation of the hot room of the Császár Baths follows a classic type, but with unique solutions. Similar playfulness[74] is not unknown in the bath architecture of the Ottoman Empire. Perhaps, it is not a coincidence that a close parallel has been found in one of Sokollu Mehmed Pasha's baths in Edirne, which was built by Mimar Sinan.[75]

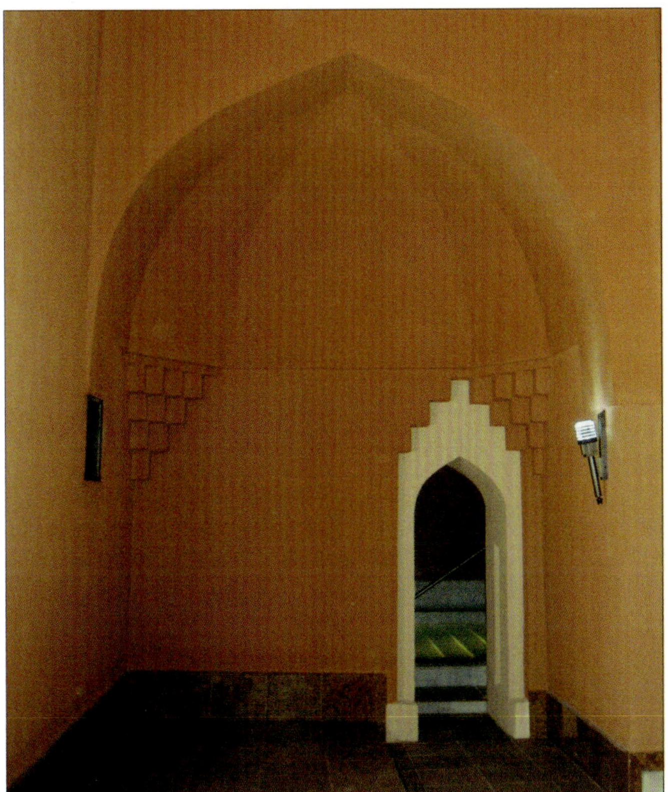

Figure 71. One of the *iwans* at the restored Császár Baths

The star-shaped hot rooms of the Rác Thermal Baths, the Király Baths in Buda, and the bath in Székesfehérvár do not belong to the most common floor plan solutions, although they were relatively popular in the 16th century. At this time, however, in most cases, a single private bath is not found in the buildings. This floor plan type was rather chosen in smaller baths such as in the first period of the Rác Thermal Baths. The characteristic solution seen at the Király Baths, where that part of the space that is divided into three is connected to the hot room in such a way as to open a private bath on both sides of the central iwan. The row of spaces is connected to the hot room with the iwan converted from one of the large niches. This solution was very widespread in the 15th century and was evident in the 16th century, too. All this strengthens the archaeological observation that the private Baths of the Rác Thermal Baths were added to the bath later because they do not constitute a unified floor plan concept. At the same time, the organisation of the Király Baths is a typical solution, the application of which can be traced back to the person of Sokollu Mustafa Pasha, who could afford to build a large bath. The Rác Thermal Baths are an Hungarian example of the star-shape plan that became increasingly common for smaller baths. The baths in Székesfehérvár are interesting among the example where double private baths (*halvets*) are connected to the hexagonal hot room. The hexagonal shape is not unknown in the 16th century, but appears more frequently among buildings from the 15th century.

The columned interior division of the Rudas Baths is among the rarest of architectural solutions, and there are hardly any buildings in this group. Two organisational categories can be formed: in one the columns, generally supporting equally proportioned cupolas, were organised in rows in the rectangular space (e.g. in Haseki Hürrem's steam bath in Istanbul[76]). In the other the columns were organised as a polygon to support a central cupola, with the space between that and the side walls being covered by other types of ceiling vaults. This latter solution reaches back to the earliest period of Ottoman bath architecture and the Eski Kaplija (Old Baths) built in Bursa in the 14th century. Eight columns can be found in both the hot and the warm room of this building that support a cupola over each room. However, the two baths in Istanbul mentioned above are much more interesting. One was built by Sultan Süleyman the Magnificent and the other by his Grand Vizier, Sokollu Mehmed Pasha. The two buildings with similar structures were designed by Mimar Sinan. A curious feature of Sokollu Mehmed Pasha's bath in Azapkapı is that its name, as mentioned earlier, is the same as the Ottoman era name for the Rudas baths: both are called *Yeshil Direkli Hamam*, that is, the Green Pillar Baths. Another similarity is that they also have asymmetrically positioned warm rooms, as do the Rudas Baths in Buda. However, the bath in Buda is much bigger than the ones in Istanbul.[77]

The three major sections (entrance hall, warm and hot rooms) rigidly follow one another in the baths in Buda. This regularity can be seen in most cases in the baths built by the Sultan and in the buildings of Mimar Sinan, too. However, it can clearly be seen on the works of the great architect that he tried to be more creative, and some unique or rarely used solutions can always be found in his buildings.[78] Architectural elements related to this architectural school also appear in the baths in Buda: on the one hand the columned Rudas Baths and on the other hand the unique hot room construction of the Császár Baths. Although the biographies of Sinan do not mention that he ever intended to build a bath in Buda, we know that he designed a *türbe* (mausoleum) there for Sokollu Mustafa Pasha and also a mosque.[79] Based on all this, the special architectural elements of the two baths mentioned above can be attributed to the influence of

Sinan if not to him personally. The Rudas, Király and Császár baths were commissioned one after the other by Mustafa Pasha. The character, choice of materials and close chronology of the buildings indicate that the workers of the same architect built them. The research of Gülru Necipoğlu[80] has shown that during this period the chief architects who worked in significant cities were in contact with the chief architect of the Empire, Mimar Sinan (*Figure 72*). The chief architect of Buda of 1572 is detailed in the accounts of the reconstruction of the mosque of Sultan Süleyman in the Buda Castle (the medieval St. Mary church building converted into a mosque). As the baths of Sokollu Mustafa Pasha were also built in this period, we can most probably connect these to the chief architect of Buda. The Pasha and his chief architect certainly consulted the chief architect of the Empire, but it can also be imagined that they got the 'plans' of the buildings in Buda straight from the Sultan's workshop.

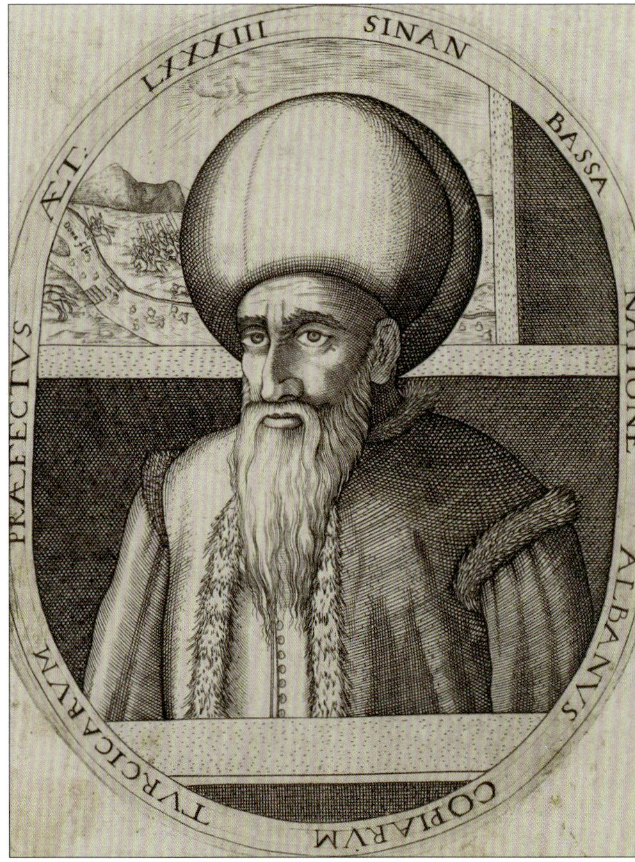

Figure 72. Portrait of Mimar Sinan, 16th century

Considering the above, it is no coincidence that clearly classic Ottoman style bath buildings appeared in the occupied territory. These are characterised by a consistent floor plan system: a rectangular space connected to a large entrance hall that is divided into several smaller warm rooms that were followed by a hot room and maybe a few private baths. Buildings were decorated moderately, typically with tripartite organisation of openings and niches, fields around the doors, changes in the plane surfaces and sparse stalactite ornamentation. The stone basins and the back panels of the wall fountains were also sparsely ornamented. Sokollu Mustafa's role as developer, meant baths were built during the occupation that were unique in the context of the Empire as a whole, and that can be confidently referred to as outstanding works of art.

VIII. The Research History of the Baths

The process of scientifically researching the Turkish baths set out from several places with architects, historians, archaeologists and art historians all engaging with it. For a long time, these scholarly researchers worked parallel to one another until, in the middle of the 20th century, the threads came together as one. Since then, the various branches of science have worked together to clarify knowledge of the structures, building solutions and significance of these edifices and, to some extent, their histories. In modern research, a complex approach and cooperation between the various disciplines is typical, and essential in the current example of 400-year-old, sometimes standing, sometimes totally ruined buildings.

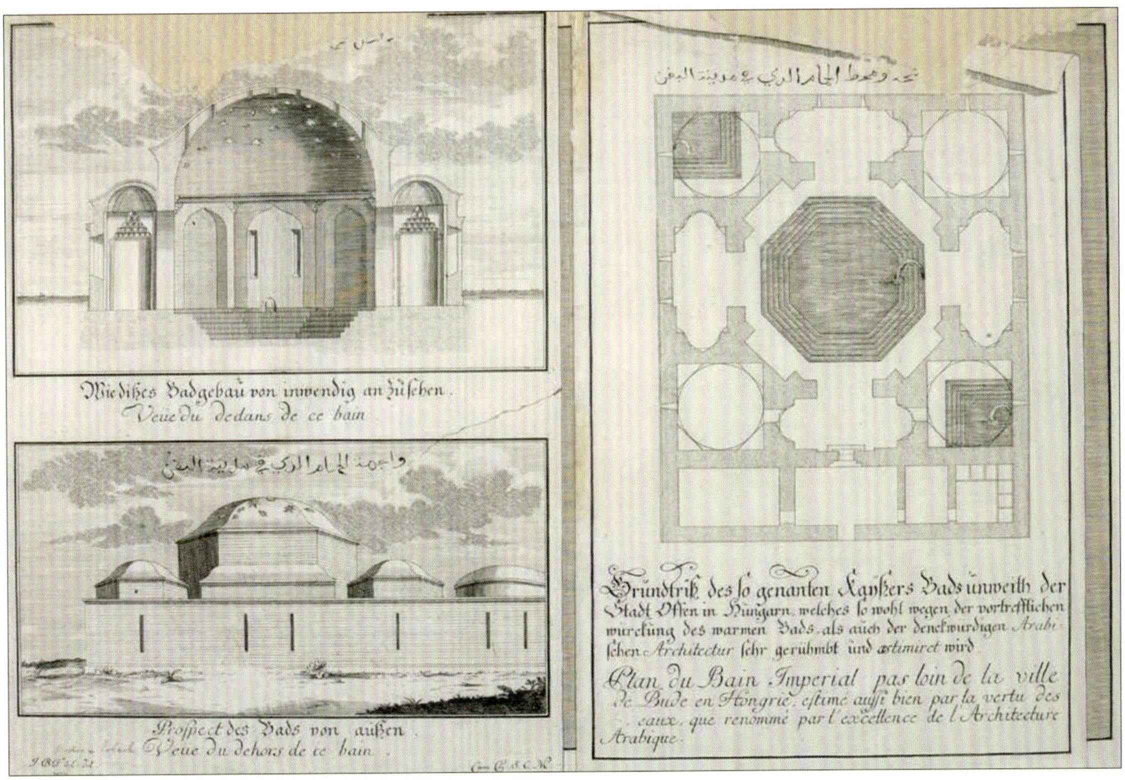

Figure 73. Drawing of the Császár Baths by Fischer von Erlach, early 18th century

The Ottoman origins of the thermal baths in Buda have never been forgotten, the Ottoman forms of parts of the buildings awoke the interest of architects very early on. At the start of the 18th century, Johann Bernhard Fischer von Erlach, an Austrian court architect, completed exploratory drawings of the Császár Baths (*Figure 73*),[81] precisely because of the eastern character of the buildings. In the 18th-19th centuries more explorations were made of bath buildings, mostly to make use of the buildings or alter them in some way (*Figure 74-75*). This is how we came to have very precise architectural planning materials on the Ferhad Pasha Baths in Pécs and the thermal baths of Buda.

Even at that time, historians were showing an interest in the subject. In 1837, Ferenc Linzbauer gathered together mediaeval and Ottoman era source materials on the baths of Buda.[82] As a doctor, Linzbauer was primarily interested in researching the medicinal history of the hot baths, but in doing so prepared a collection on the Ottoman remains. At the end of the 19th century Árpád Károlyi made a comparison between the appearances of the baths in Ottoman era written sources and today's extant buildings.[83]

Scientific interest sharpened in the 20th century, and the generally accepted viewpoint among experts became that these structures deserved to be included among the protected historic buildings of Hungary. So it was that the

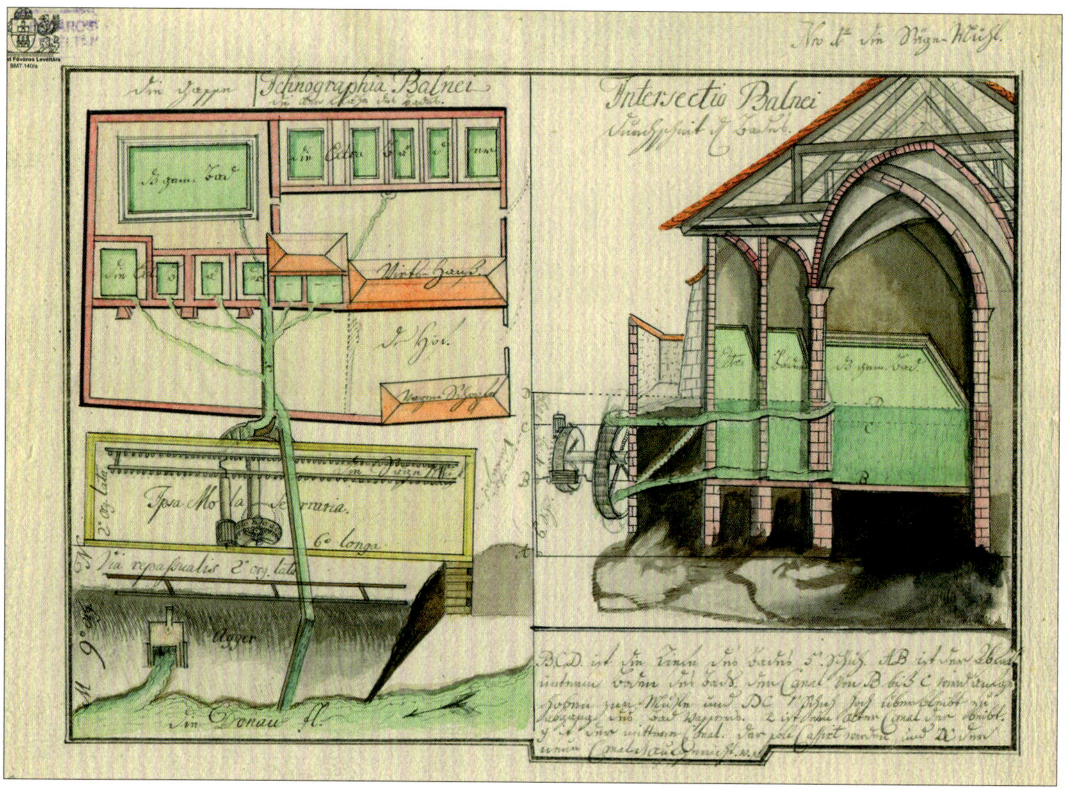

Figure 74. Plan of the sawmill built beside the Rudas Baths in the 18th century, 1712

architects also explored the Ottoman buildings (in 1917 under the direction of Ernő Foerk, the notable architect and church builder),[84] later József Molnár experimented in locating the standing bath buildings of the Ottoman era.[85] While this work was being done, the esteemed expert on the Ottomans, Lajos Fekete, was trying to confirm the Ottoman era buildings in Buda.[86] He analysed the written data, the surviving pictorial depictions and the known buildings to identify the extant buildings represented by their Ottoman era names. At that time, he referred to the sources on the baths as chaotic, and we certainly do in fact know many more names of baths than we do actual bath buildings.

It was at this time that the first parts of the ruined Ottoman era steam baths came to light in Pest during construction at the Piarist Grammar School (1914), and in Pécs during the laying of drains (1927). Both these examples show that spectacular ruins are hidden in the ground beneath the buildings of modern towns, and not only ruins from mediaeval Hungary, but also from the Ottoman period. In the early period of Hungarian archaeology, the first research on the Ottoman era took place; thus, Ottó Szőnyi's excellent analysis of the baths in Pécs could be supported by an analysis of the 18th century architectural explorations.

With all these results, the researchers and architects of the era became aware of the value of the bath buildings. Due to this fact, in the 1930s, when the houses of the Tabán district in Buda were demolished, the Rác Baths were left untouched. The oriental character and long history of the thermal baths of Buda had become an asset.

The restoration of the damaged bathing facilities following the devastation of the Second World War provided Győző Gerő, a Turkologist and archaeologist, with an opportunity to research the buildings. He can be regarded as the founder of Ottoman archaeology in the modern sense in Hungary, who was as comfortable in the methodology of building archaeology as he was in researching the material culture of the past or understanding contemporaneous historical sources. On large surfaces, he first worked on the Király Baths (1955),[87] and in tandem with his work, a structural survey and research into the buildings were also carried out. It was exceedingly fortunate that in the same year, using archaeological methods, he discovered and excavated the Beylerbey of Buda Baths. A few years later, in 1958, he found the Eger Baths and began the excavation of this building that continued over many years. Through his work, the Memi Pasha Baths in Pécs and the Toygun Pasha Baths in Buda were also excavated. As a specialist he helped his colleagues István Horváth and Gyula Siklósi at Fehervár and Esztergom, who were also researching bath buildings using archaeological methods. All this resulted in a whole series of Turkish baths being excavated in the latter part of the 20th Century. Initially, József Molnár presented them in a minor promotional work,[88] and then Győző Gerő, in his book on the Ottoman architecture in Hungary, also mentioned these buildings from the era of Ottoman occupation.[89]

At the beginning of the 21st century, due to the modernization of functional baths and numerous construction projects, research into operating baths and reburied bath ruins could be carried out. I personally led these excavations in Buda, and I was able to contribute to those that took place on the Pest side. The recent research has been the inspiration for the release of this book. In addition to archaeological excavations, historical research has also taken on new impetus: Balázs Sudár[90] has gathered together the data on the baths from the era of the Ottoman occupation.

Since the 19th century, in the light of increasingly significant research, an especially important question has confronted each generation of researchers: what should be done with the exposed buildings? In the case of functioning buildings, the question became one of how the architect and the investor can use the results of archaeological excavations, and of how much of an opportunity exists to restore the systems and character of the Ottoman era building. There were a variety of different responses to these questions in the case of the thermal baths of Buda.

The dilemma between presentation or reburial came to the fore in the instance of excavated ruins. The fates of these buildings have varied. The relatively weather-proof example of restoration in Pécs compared to against decades of dereliction in Eger where the ruins can now be visited only under dry conditions, meaning those baths can finally be listed among the more acceptable solutions. In sharp contrast the is the alarming fate of the Fehervár Baths, which are in a constantly declining state of dilapidation. Unfortunately, the Pest baths excavated at the start of the 21st century was reburied rather than the option of its presentation being chosen.

In the next part of this volume you can read individually the stories of these Hungarian buildings and witness what has become of them today. We will also present, with the help of the archaeological research tools and the documentation made during the excavations, the varied architectural solutions, some of which are fabulous, that are no longer visible or have been destroyed in the meantime. In this way we can help those who visit the buildings currently used as baths to discover the Ottoman era detail and architectural solutions. In their current condition Hungary's Ottoman baths present the architecture of the empire, the work of the research disciplines and the elements of a living bath culture that has been in existence for centuries.

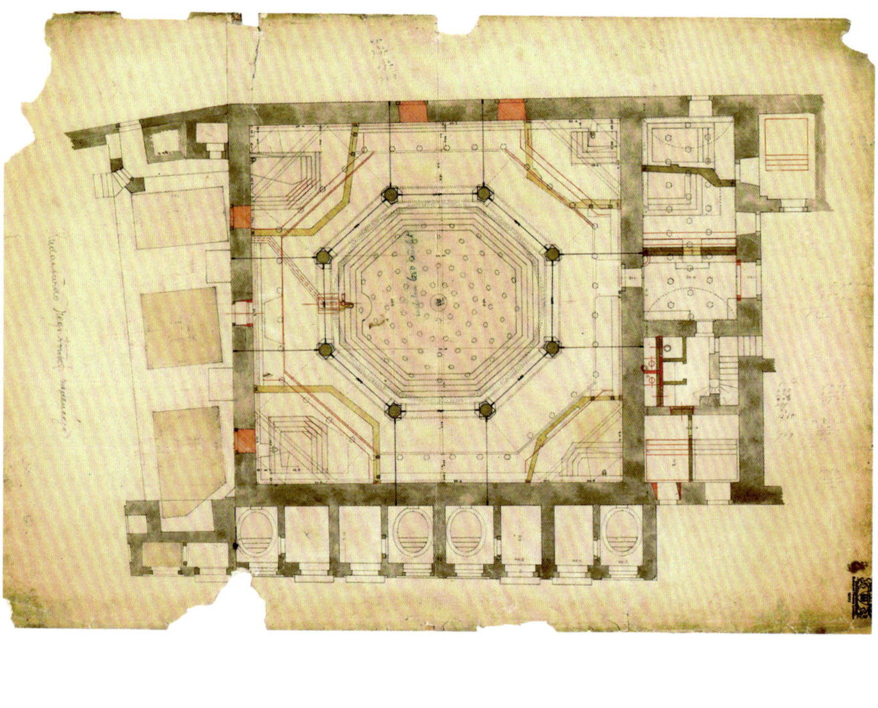

Figure 75. The 19th-century plan for rebuilding the Rudas Baths

IX. Introduction to the Architectural Remains of the Turkish Bath Buildings of Hungary

Turkish baths operating in Hungary today

The Rudas Baths, Buda

Budapest I., Döbrentei tér 9.

The most imposing of the Turkish baths that remain in Hungary (*Figure* 76), they were considered special even in the Ottoman era because of their column structure and the enormous size of the hot room (*Figure* 77). The remaining hot and warm rooms of the Turkish baths are embraced by the 18th and 19th century parts of the building. Today, it is one of the most renowned baths in Budapest.

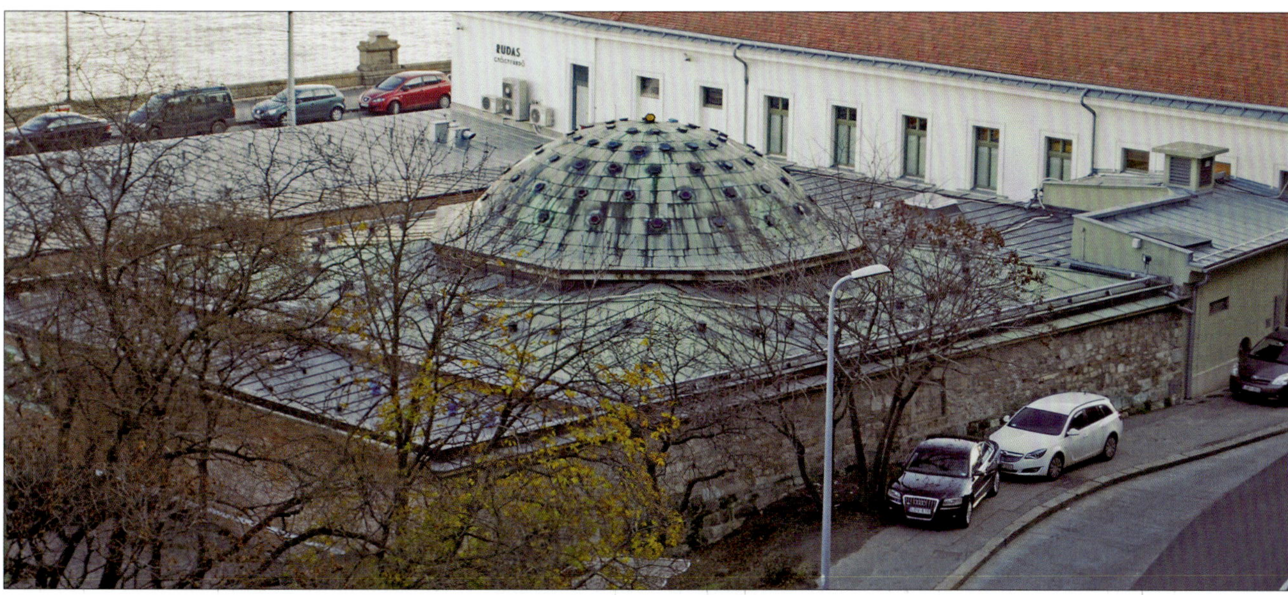

Figure 76. The Rudas Baths in Buda

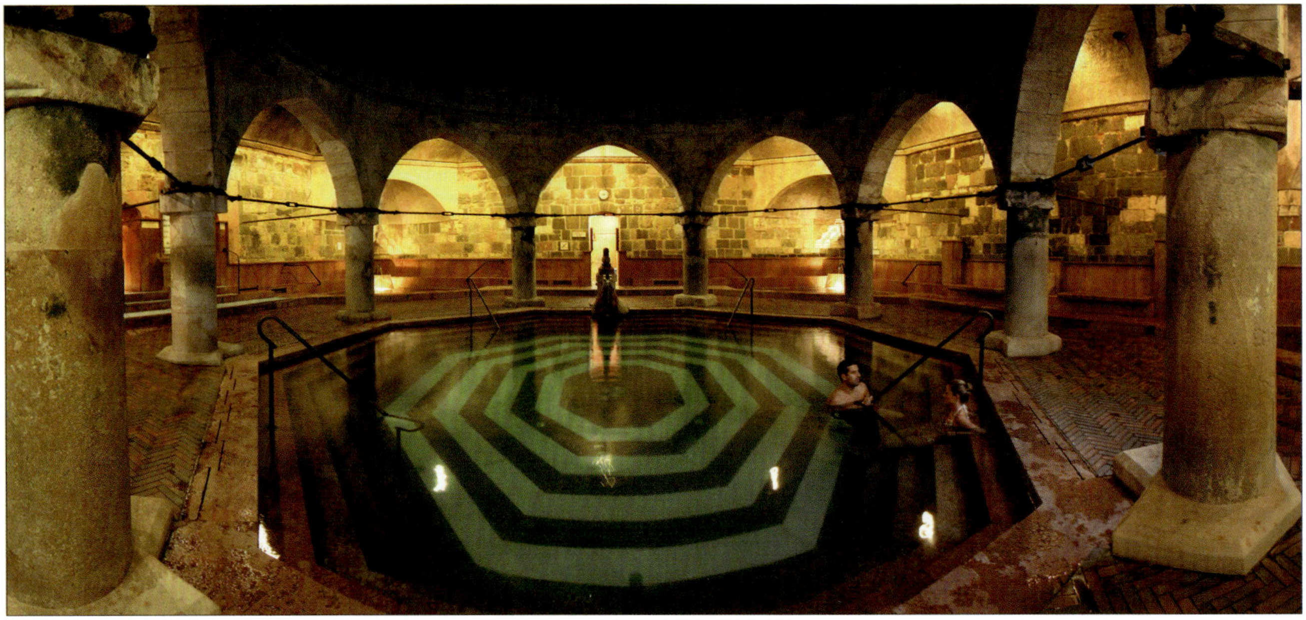

Figure 77. Panoramic view of the eight columns in the hot room of the restored Rudas Baths

Founder:	Sokollu Mustafa Pasha
Year founded:	1571/1572
Ottoman era name:	*Yeshil Direkli Ilija* (Green Pillar Baths)
Type:	thermal baths
Ground plan type:	pillared hot room (G type) (*Figure 78*)
Directors of excavation:	Sándor Garády, Adrienn Papp
Excavation date:	1937 (Sándor Garády), 2004-2005 (Adrienn Papp)
Publications:	Lászay-Papp 2004; Lászay-Papp 2005; Lászay-Papp 2006; Lászay-Papp 2009, pp. 291-297; Papp-Grynaeus 2011

HISTORY

In the Ottoman era they were known as *Yeshil Direkli Ilija* (Green Pillar Baths).[91] Franciscus Omichius[92] mentions them in 1572 as the baths beneath Gellért Hill, and states that the pasha (Sokollu Mustafa) built the dome. The foundation of Sokollu Mustafa Pasha records that he had them built. The precise date of the building was determined as 1571/72 through dendrochronological examination of the excavated wooden posts.[93]

The baths stood in an area that was built over in the Middle Ages, so unravelling its history began with the excavation of the medieval buildings on the site.[94] The new bath was constructed between the main road and the Danube, with its entrance on the northern side. During the excavations, a single piece of Ottoman era construction was discovered: the large dimensions of the building meant there had been no need for expansion, but the remains of Ottoman service work could be explored.[95]

Written records state that during the war of reconquest the baths were not damaged,[96] however, the entrance hall was portrayed in a drawing from 1712,[97] as being in a courtyard. In fact, there are reports that as early as 1699 the rooms on the bath courtyard were covered with a dome.[98] This suggests that during the conflict the building was damaged: that is, the dome over the entrance hall collapsed to create a courtyard around which various rooms were later built onto its walls. This condition is shown in drawings from 1832 by the architect József Dankó Jnr (see *Figure 31*).[99]

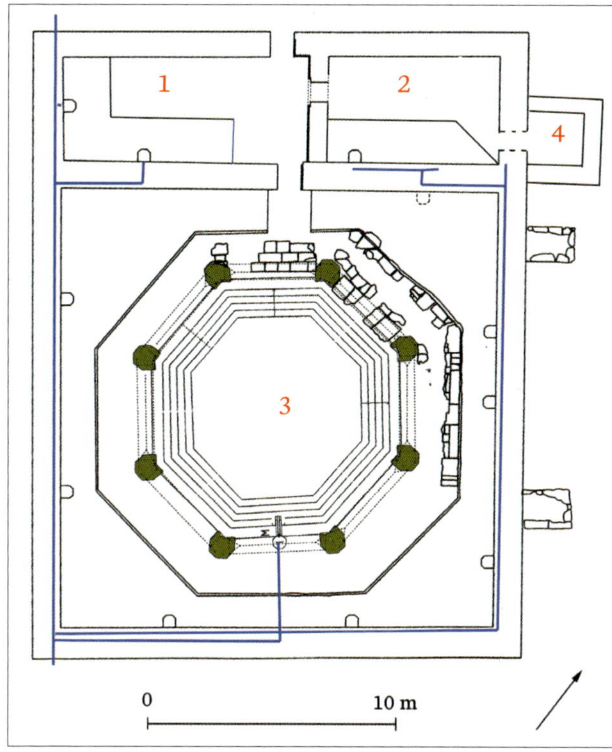

Figure 78. Floorplan of the Rudas Baths. 1-2. Warm areas. 3. Hot area. 4. Toilet

The bath came into the ownership of the capital in 1696 and has been in continual ownership since then. Several design contests and a committee meeting report for reconstruction track the history of the building.[100]

The first detailed drawings of the baths were made in 1712 in reference to the neighbouring mill buildings (see *Figure 74*).[101] Fewer than 30 years after the reconquest of the city, the institution was significantly developed: new swimming pools were constructed in the former entrance hall area and in the hot room. Renovation of the very well-preserved baths was carried out in 1794–1795, but to what manner and degree we do not know.[102]

The 19th-century changes are easier to follow, as we have several series of plans from this century. The area of the Ottoman entrance hall functioned as a courtyard until the expansion of the building in 1880. The eastern wall was demolished in 1831 during building works. At that time the area between the buttresses on the east and south walls was built in. By the mid-19th century the metal struts between the pillars that supported the dome had been destroyed, they were already absent from Rudolf Alt's drawing from 1860.

The first major extension of the baths was completed in the 1880s to plans by Miklós Ybl; however, in these the Ottoman era elements were not significantly altered. The first step was the adaption of the Ottoman era entrance hall. At the same time, the Ottoman era warm areas were also refurbished.[103] It was then that the main entrance door to the

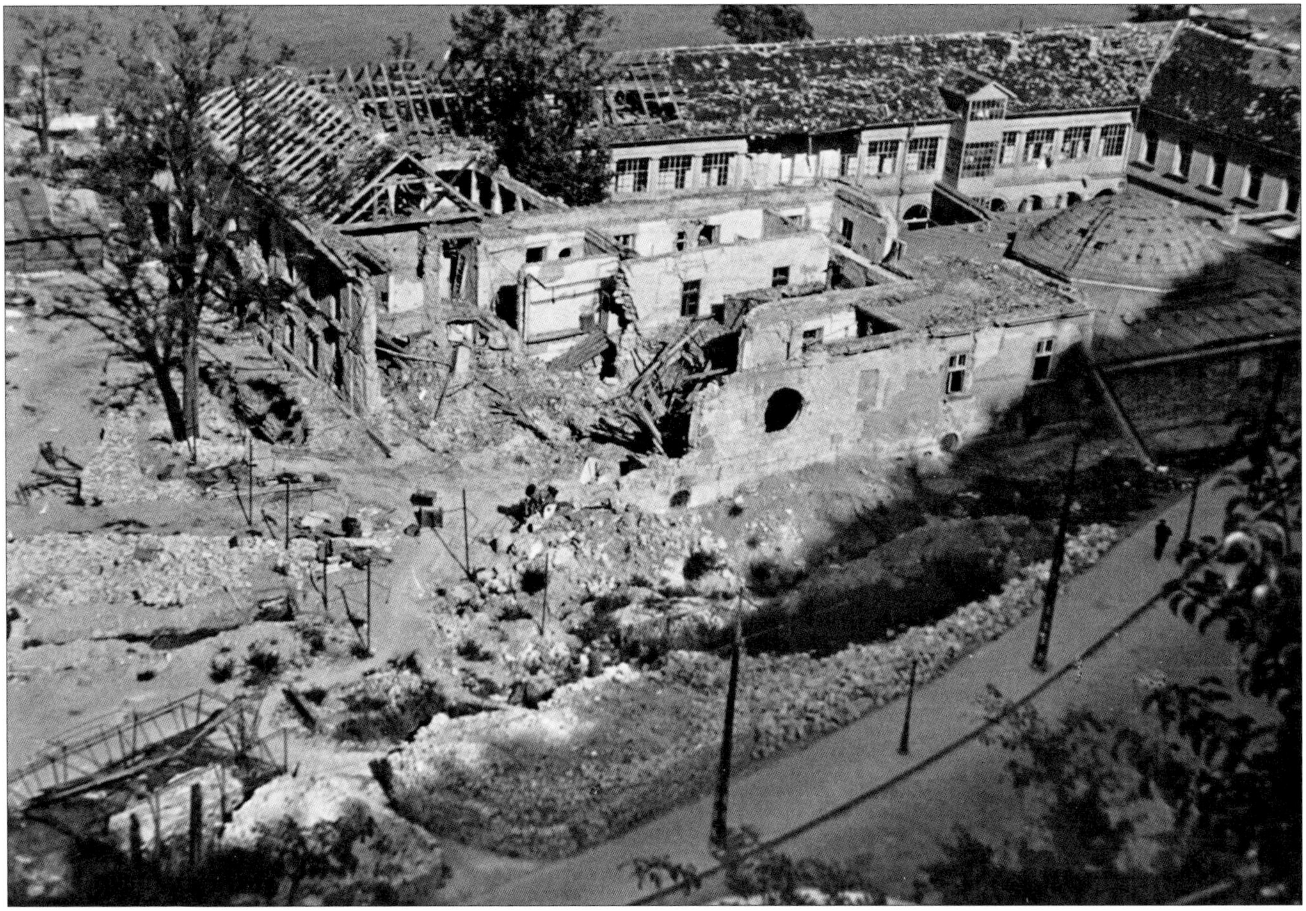

Figure 79. The Rudas Baths following damage inflicted during the Second World War

area beneath the dome was widened and the barrel vaulted arrangement created that exists today: the asymmetrical design was replaced by a symmetrical one, and a stone frame, probably from the Ottoman era, was set into the new wall. The variously sized and shaped corner enclosures in the hot rooms were regularized and the windows were walled up.[104]

At the beginning of the 20th century, modification of the obsolete bath-tub parts of the building was planned, but this major construction was postponed because of the outbreak of the First World War. During the Second World War, the northern part of the baths were damaged most (*Figure 79*), and were then dismantled during post-war reconstruction. It was at this time that the Ottoman era hall of the baths was removed. The baths' remaining thermal area was explored in 2004–2005 (*Figure 80*).

DESCRIPTION OF THE BUILDING

Research[105] was carried out during the refurbishment of the thermal part of the Rudas Baths. In accordance with the prepared design plans, the depths of the domed space were excavated while in the space beneath the barrel vaulting there was minimal probing and the surface beneath the new cladding could be opened up. The baths were parallel to the Danube, lying northwest-southeast,[106] the entrance was on the northwest side. There are currently two tracts: the warm rooms on the north and the hot room south of them.

The entrance hall

The entrance hall was destroyed, its size and location is recorded by 19th-century architectural surveys. It was nearly as large as the hot room, with its entrance on the north side. The wall thickness on the plans is the same as the thickness of the spine discovered during archaeological research. According to this, the walls of the building were 90 centimetres thick. They would not have been able to support a dome with a diameter of nearly 18 meters, so there would have been either a cupola or a wooden ceiling covering the entrance hall as in the hot room. Some details of the northern walls are known from the excavations by Sándor Garády who explored the northern edge of the baths before the Second World War.

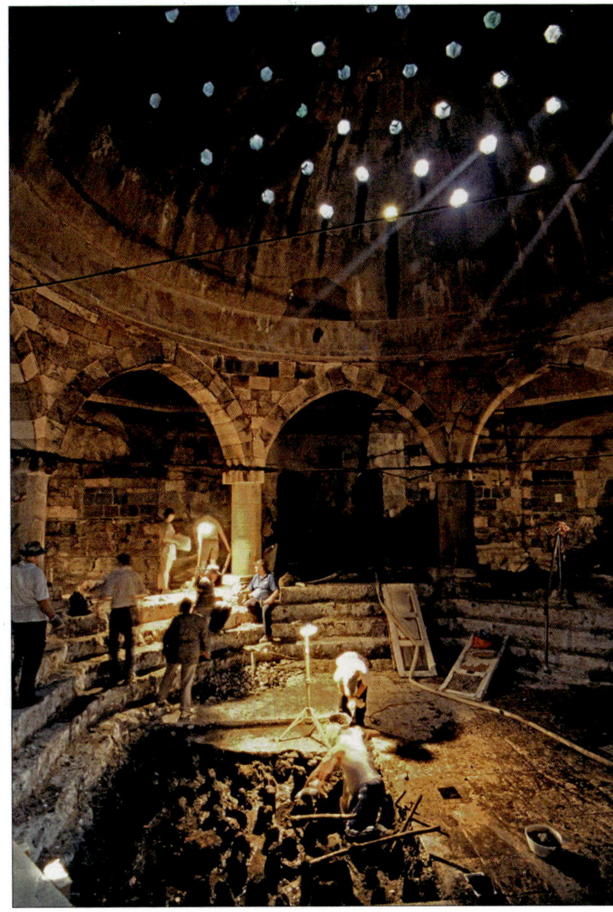

Figure 80. The Ottoman era wooden posts beneath the basin of the hot room at the Rudas Baths

The warm areas

In the Ottoman era there were two warm rooms, the step patterned doorway to the smaller eastern area remains even today (*Figures 81-82*). The western room is currently divided in two by a brick wall. The floors of these areas were destroyed when modern pools were created here, leaving only fragmentary information to be gleaned from the ground plan. What is certain is that in the Ottoman era there were no pools in the warm rooms, but by the walls there were stone curb benches. The presence of benches and water fountains can be determined by the water pipes remaining in the walls. The western room was expanded by two niches that were formed during a later conversion.

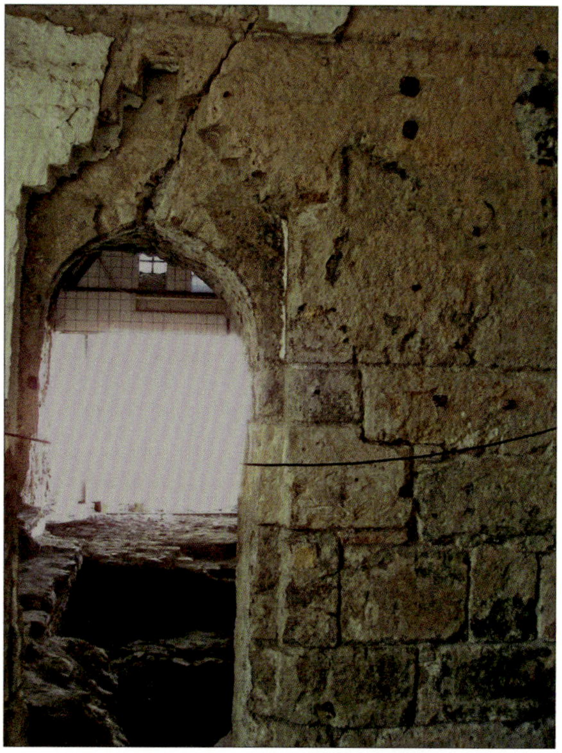

Figure 81. Stepped ornamentation of the door between the warm rooms at the Rudas Baths during excavation

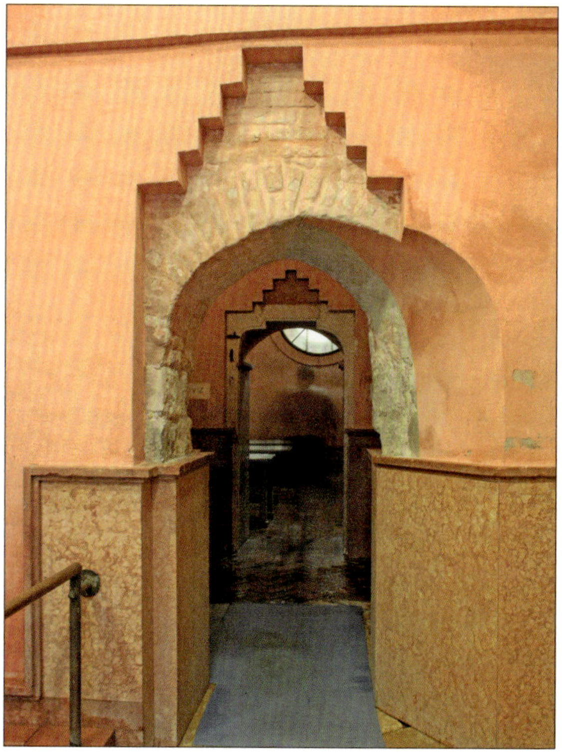

Figure 82. Stepped ornamentation of the doorway between the warm rooms at the Rudas Baths following reconstruction

The rooms are covered with barrel vaults with hexagonal skylights. There was no window in the west room, and the eastern facade wall has not survived, but it is unlikely that there was a window as the toilet was on the outside.

The toilet

The toilet opened from the east warm room and lay outside the main building. The north side wall and the drainage channel were also exposed.

The hot room

This is the most interesting space among the Ottoman buildings of Hungary (*Figure 83*). Eight pillars support the central dome, which are surrounded by barrel vaulting. In the corners beneath the cloister arches stalactite ornaments hang. By the wall the octagonal pool sides are lined with benches. A section of the original flooring was uncovered that enabled a good reconstruction. There were no pools in the corners in the Ottoman era. The original white limestone steps to the Ottoman era pool that lies at the centre of the room remain although their coverings were missing at the time of excavation. The former paving and the sub-pool pillar system were demolished, which were also suited to dendrochronological examination and based on which it was possible to date precisely the construction of the baths (see *Figure 80*).

The ceramic water pipes in the walls survived in good condition, into which system stone elements were set into the wall to create water fountains. The pool was filled by a separate pipe which was a lot thicker than those in the water fountain system.

On the walls, small areas of residual plaster were also excavated. The hall's real attractions are the pillars, one of which is not original. According to Edward Brown, an English physician,[107] it is clear that at the end of the Ottoman era the columns of the hot room were connected with iron struts, but it is unclear whether that was the case when they were constructed or whether it was something that was required later.

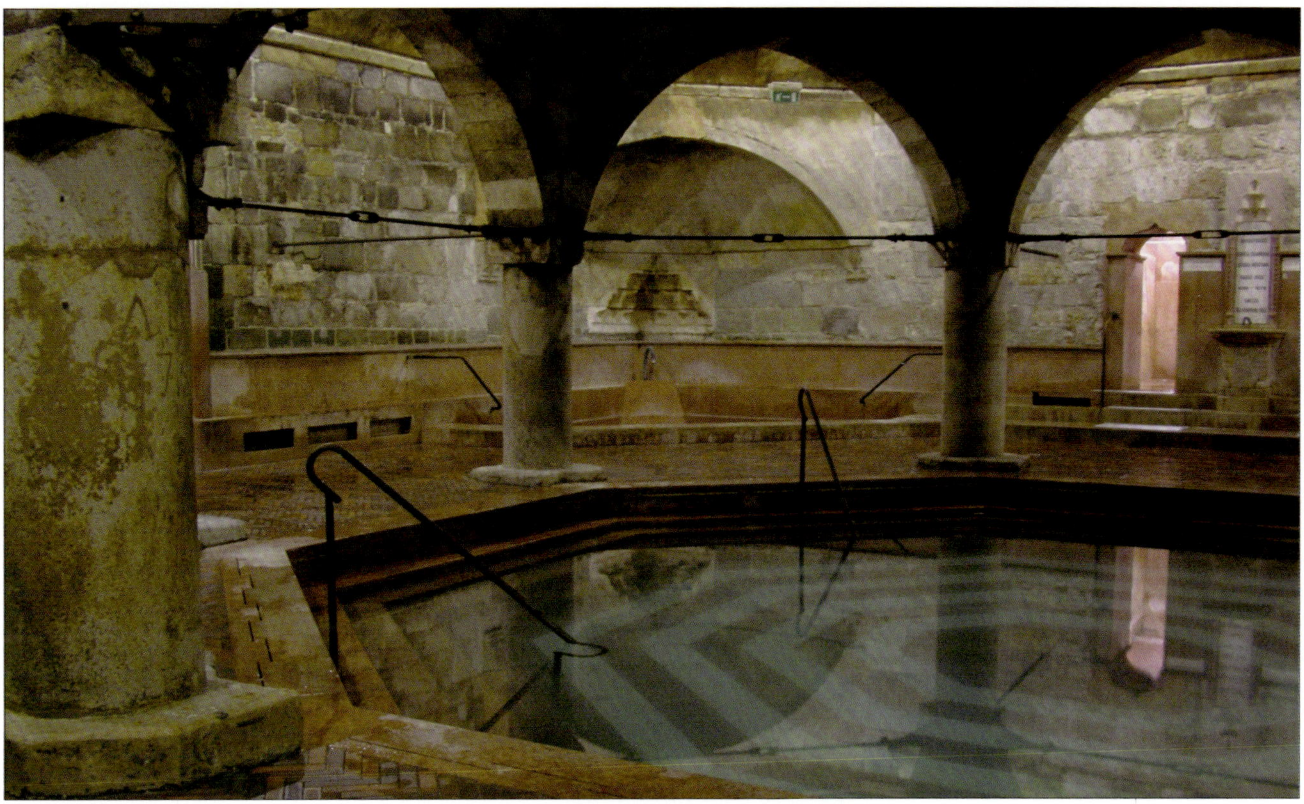

Figure 83. Interior of the Rudas Baths today

The Császár Baths, Buda

Budapest II., Árpád fejedelem útja 7.

The Császár Baths (The Emperor's Baths) also won the admiration of Ottoman travellers for their scale and layout. Today it is only the hot room that remains, and that is barely noticeable among all the hospital buildings (*Figure 84*). During the last period of construction, in the 1970s, the last remnants of the warm room and the foyer of the baths were demolished. At that time Győző Gerő documented the Ottoman remains that came to light. The interior and the immediate surroundings of the building were explored through archaeological excavations.

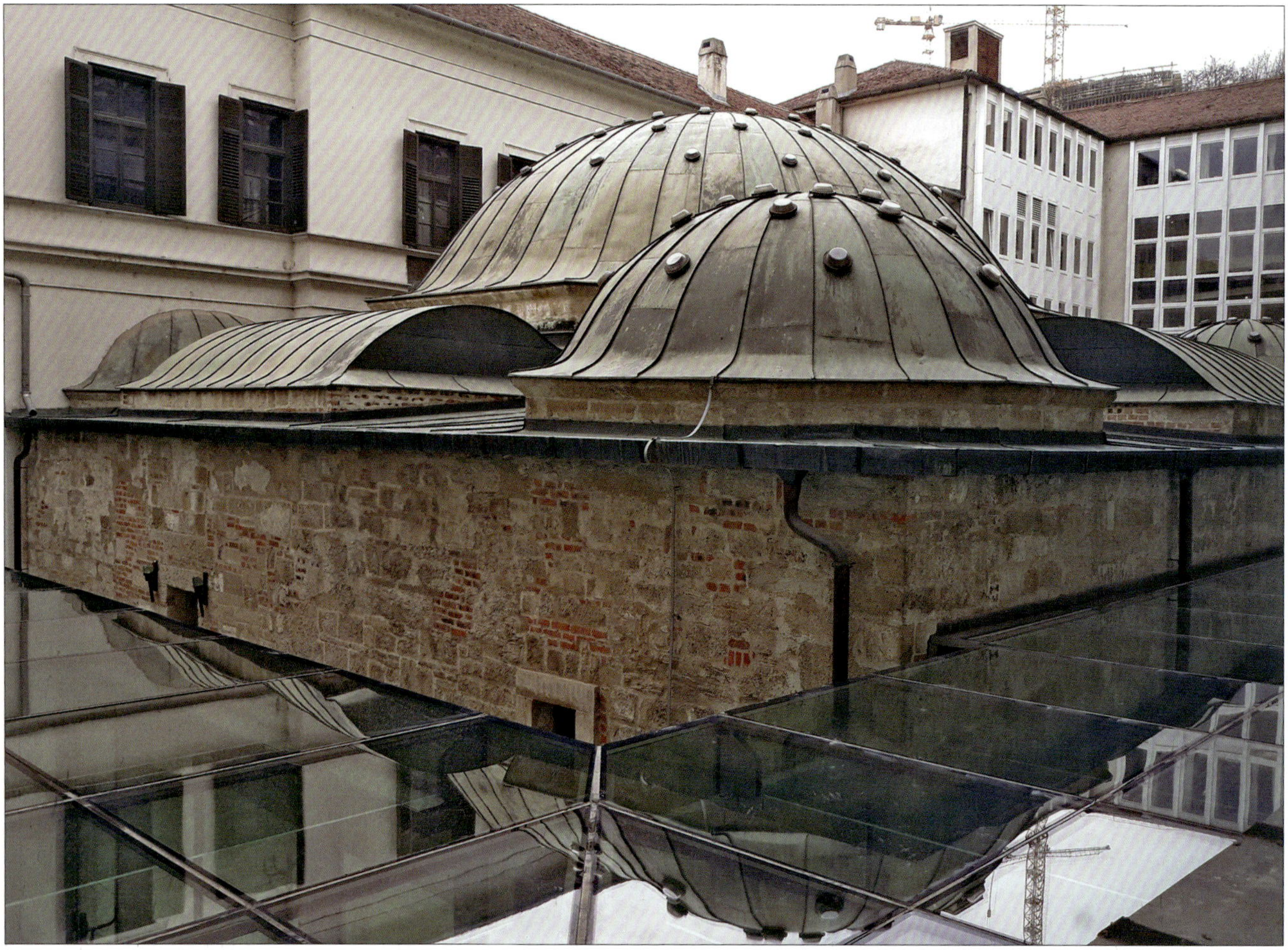

Figure 84. The domes over the Császár Baths, Buda

Founded by:	Sokollu Mustafa Pasha
Year of founding:	1574
Ottoman era name:	*Veli Bey Ilijasi* (Veli Bey Baths)
Type:	thermal bath
Ground plan type:	cross formation (A type) group variation (*Figure 88*)
Director of excavation:	Adrienn Papp
Date of excavation:	2008-2009
Publications:	GERŐ 1980, pp. 103-106; LÁSZAY-PAPP 2007; LÁSZAY-PAPP 2008; LÁSZAY-PAPP 2009, pp. 302-309; PAPP-LÁSZAY 2009-2010; PAPP-GRYNAEUS 2011

HISTORY

The baths belong among the very few Ottoman buildings in Hungary whose founding inscription has been preserved (*Figure 85*).[108] Nowadays we have a reproduction, a painted graphic copy, of the text of the story—since destroyed—that Balázs Sudár analysed in order to reconstruct the baths. Included in this inscription was the year of the building's construction, according to Ottoman custom, somewhat concealed, but matching the date determined through a dendrochronological study of excavated posts:[109] the bath was built in 1574 by Sokollu Mustafa Pasha. It is, therefore, a little surprising that the institution was named Veli Bey Baths in Ottoman times - from which the modern name is derived: Veli Bey Baths. Why this name should have been given to or stuck to the baths has never been satisfactorily resolved, nor the relationship between the Veli Bey and the Császár Baths.

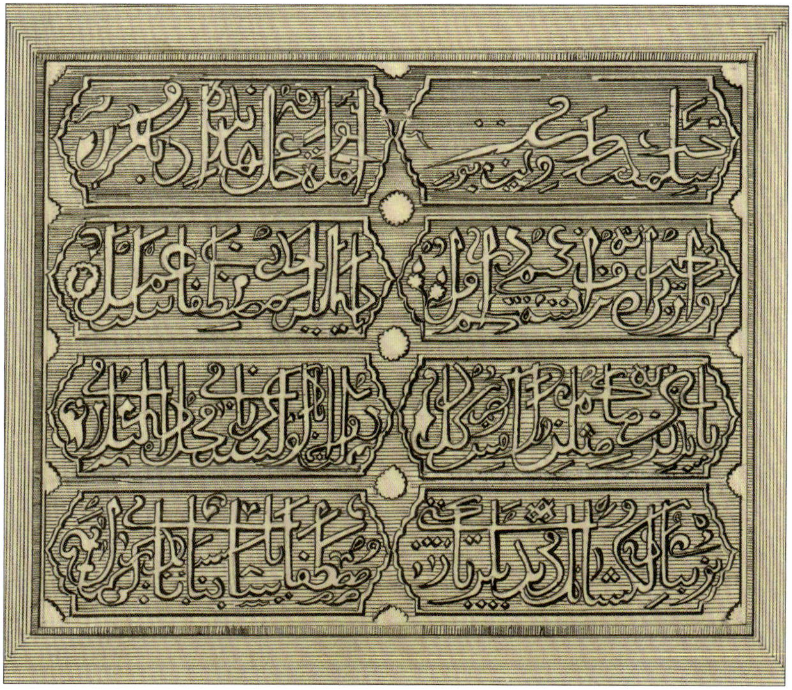

Figure 85. Engraving taken from a drawing made by Lipót Sztankovits of Sokollu Mustafa's dedication board of the Császár Baths, 1574

Only a small part of the bath survived from which a single piece of Ottoman era construction can be seen. However, several signs of service also surfaced. Fortunately, in the modern age the Ottoman plaster was not entirely removed, so it was possible to examine it across a relatively large surface.

One interesting piece of evidence for the use of the bath after the Ottoman era was found in the north-eastern corner of the room, where the water pipes used by the Turks were placed in the walls had in one section been repaired with an 18th-century water pipe. This suggests that even after the Ottoman era the earlier pipes were used, and during maintenance only the defective section was replaced.

We know little of the 18th-century history of the baths, their new golden age and, in connection with that, their era of major reconstruction was in the 19th century. János Lipszky[110] preserved a snapshot of their 18th-century condition in his map. The manner in which the baths are depicted as somewhat strange, because the shape of a cupola room is marked as a circle. Certainly, the interior design could have led to this false representation. Apart from that, the map faithfully records the fact that new additions to the Ottoman building were not yet in situ. It is, however, clear that the

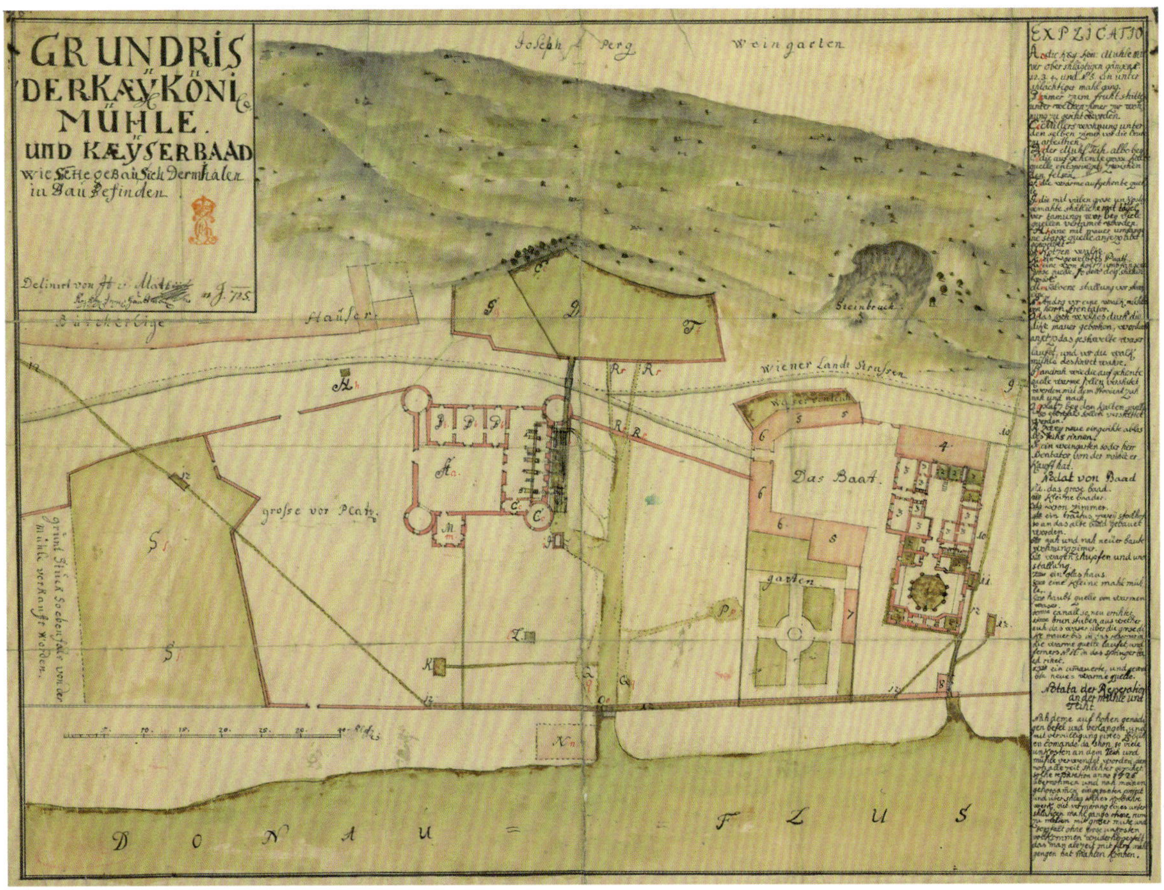

Figure 86. The Császár Baths and neighbourhood from a survey drawing of the gunpowder mill with four corner towers from 1725

entrance hall area had become a courtyard, and while its walls were lined with covered rooms, its centre lay open. Accordingly, the former roof had already collapsed and, as with other baths, the space was then used as a courtyard (*Figure 86*).

In 1802, István Marczibányi purchased the bath and donated it to the Hospitaller Order, and thus began the new age of the baths' construction. The large-scale reconstruction took place in the 1840s and 1860s, the bathing area increased considerably, but its central Ottoman era core was basically unharmed. The great demolitions took place after the Second World War, between 1960 and 1980.[111] The unfortunate demolition of the Turkish entrance hall and the temporary rooms occurred in the 1970s when the new hospital wing was built. The restoration work was accompanied by Győző Gerő's research.

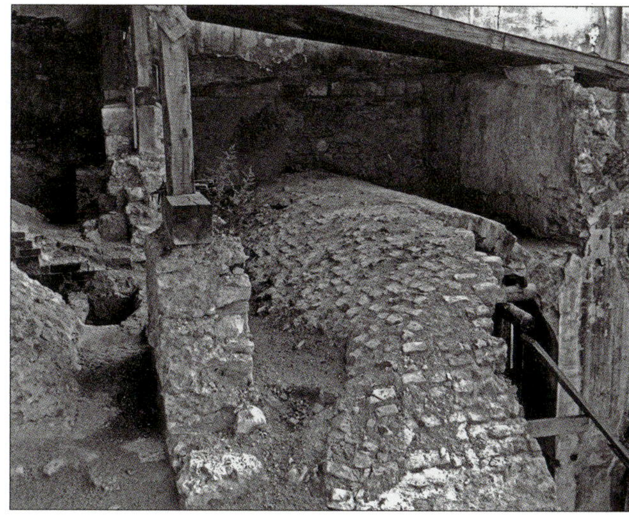

Figure 87. The now demolished vault of the warm rooms at the Császár Baths, 1974

DESCRIPTION OF THE BUILDING

Renovation of the building and the inbuilding of its immediate surroundings resulted in the baths being researched. In the Ottoman era, the bath was located between the Danube and the main road leading to Buda, on the southern side of the lake, which was fed by springs at the foot of the hill.

The entrance hall

The entrance hall was demolished in the 1970's. No documentation was made during the demolition. Its size and location are recorded in the 18th-century drawings that depict the building and its surroundings. In these an entrance hall somewhat wider than the hot room can be seen. The thickness of the wall is also indicated in the drawing, so it is probably not a large dome but rather a timber-framed ceiling. The entrance of the bath opened from the south even by 1725, in the direction of the

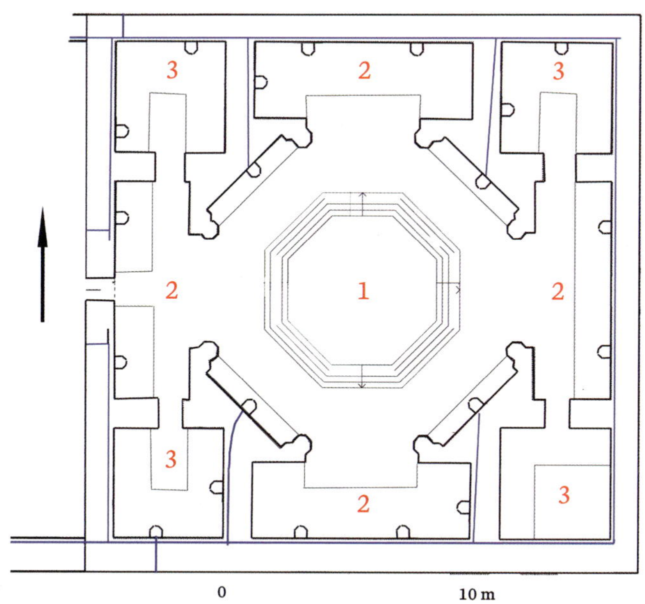

Figure 88. The floorplan for the Császár Baths (the entrance hall and the warm room were demolished). 1. Hot room. 2. *Iwans.* 3. Private baths

gunpowder mill. This is a little surprising because the main north-south road lay in front of the west wall of the bath, from where the building would have opened. Since these drawings were made a few decades after the wars of reconquest, but before the large-scale reconstructions, they can be given most credit for showing the state of the baths in the Ottoman era. An archaeological examination of the entrance to the building on the south could help to clarify this question.

The warm area

The warm area was divided into two parts but extended the full width of the hot room. In the Second World War, it was significantly damaged, and it was demolished in the 1970s when almost 80% of the domed section of the south-eastern part was still standing. During the research conducted by Győző Gerő, a survey was carried out of the bath ceiling which was then exposed from under the baroque roof (*Figure 87*).

The hot room

The hot room is the most beautifully preserved room of the baths, with an octagonal pool in the centre (see *Figure 88*) above which a dome was raised. In the corners there were private baths, and the rectangular spaces between them were individually made up of two *iwans*, each of which was closed by a cloister arch and barrel vaulting. The pool floor and the lower part of the basin were preserved in their original condition. Only a few stones from the floor and foundation of the bench running along the walls remained over a relatively small surface area. In the iwans (east and west), from where the entrance to the *halvets*—the private baths—had been opened, the bench just ran along the outer edge of the room and was adapted to become the door leading to the private baths. In the northern and southern iwans, the modern era rebuilding was so extensive that not even the foundations to the floor remained. Here we can only suppose that the benches turned alongside the shorter walls.

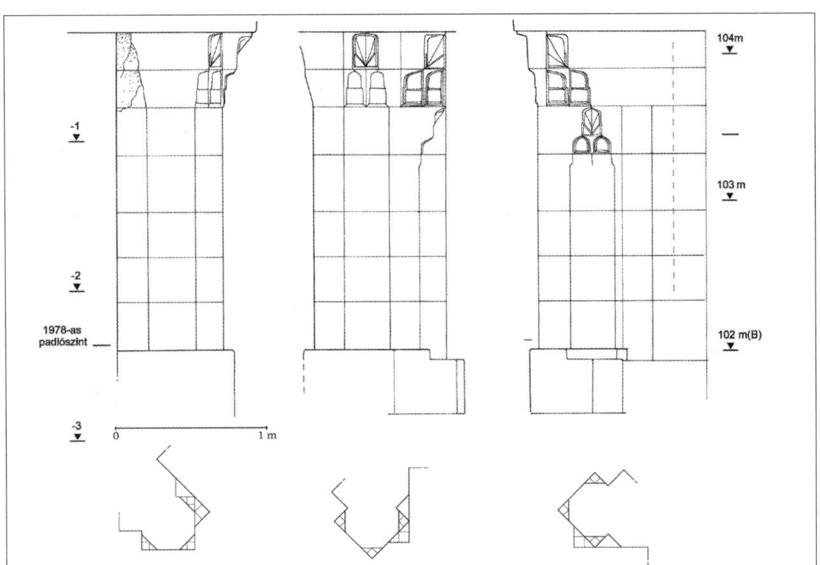

Figure 89. The survey drawing of the pillars around the hot room pool at the Császár Baths, 2007

The walls were plastered: pink, red and white plaster was exposed.[112] Two periods of coloration of the baths could be distinguished, one with the side walls

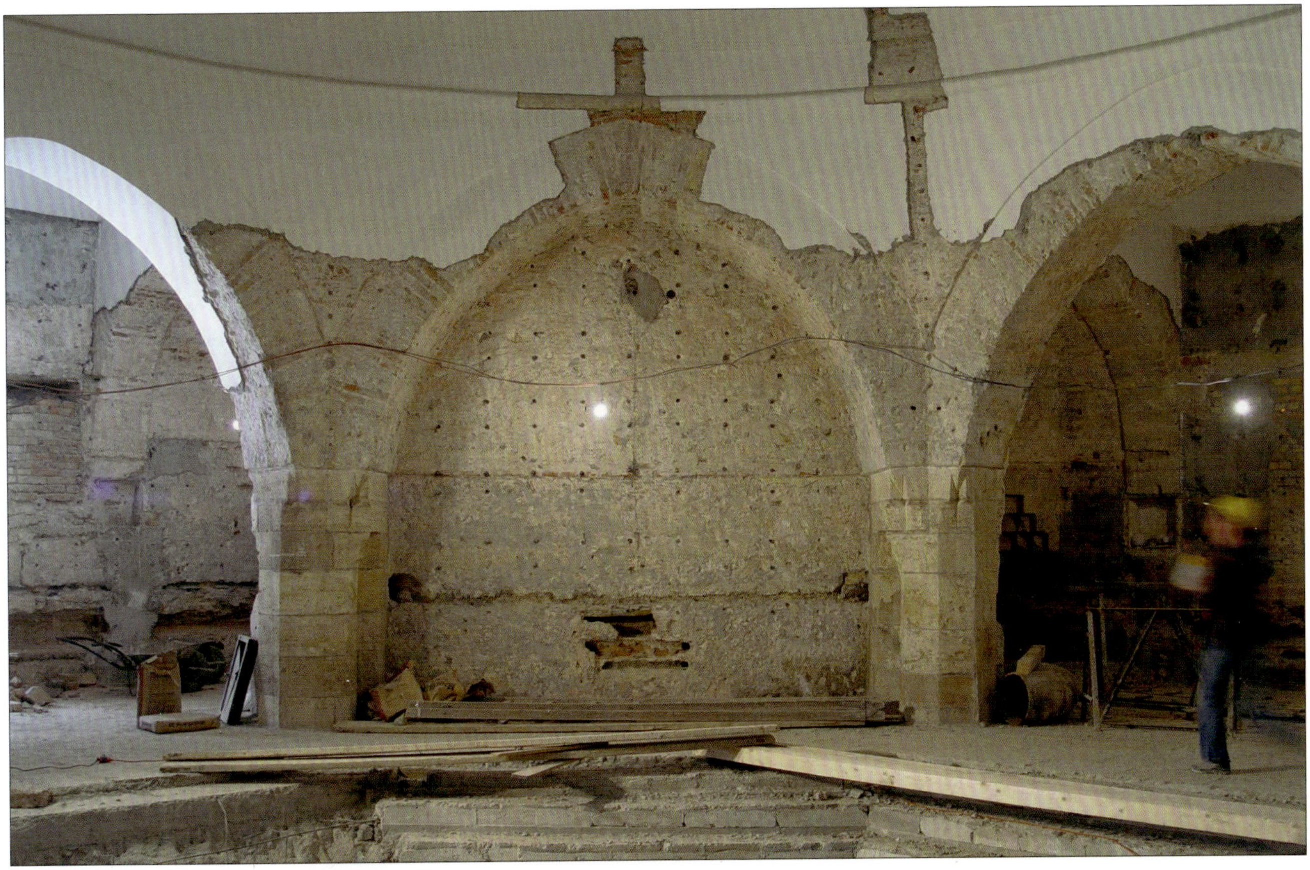

Figure 90. The Császár Baths during the excavation of the hot room

red and the vaults covered with pink plaster, later the lower part of the sidewalls were red, and the upper part and the vaults were white. More artistic are the edges of the pillars that form the sides of the large niches around the pool where cut back edges dominate (*Figures 89–90*). According to written sources, water was poured into the basin from lion-shaped ornaments, but the archaeological excavation found no evidence of that. The corners of the iwan were decorated with stalactite ornaments (*Figure 91*). In the north and south side sections decoration was imbedded into the plane, and in the western and eastern parts, the decoration stood proud of the plane. The recesses were made of stone, the projections were brick-masonry, and some were plastered over. These ornaments are made from simple cuboid shapes.

Hexagonal skylights were set in concentric circles in the vaults (the bottom line currently visible on the cupola is not original) They were in rows in the trough vaulting but arranged in groups on the barrel vaulting (see *Figure 68*).

Private baths

In each of the four corners of the hot room a small square area was built and operated as a private bath. We know from Evliya Chelebi that a pool was located in one of them. The modern age alterations have left no trace of that but based on the plaster prints on the walls we think that this pool might have been in the south-eastern private bath. In the southwestern hall, the foundations of the original floor, the Ottoman filling layers and a modern pool were discovered during the excavation. The northern side was also greatly disturbed, where once the curb benches stretched along the walls upon which fountains were set. The location of the fountains can be deduced from the remnants of the plumbing system.

Around the southern side of the bath, water tanks and water pipes were discovered (*Figure 92*), and a well was located. From this the whole system that these parts represent cannot be reconstructed, but it is certain that several smaller containers must have supplied the basins and operated the fountains. In a special way cold and warm water was used, so two types of water could be drained from the taps.

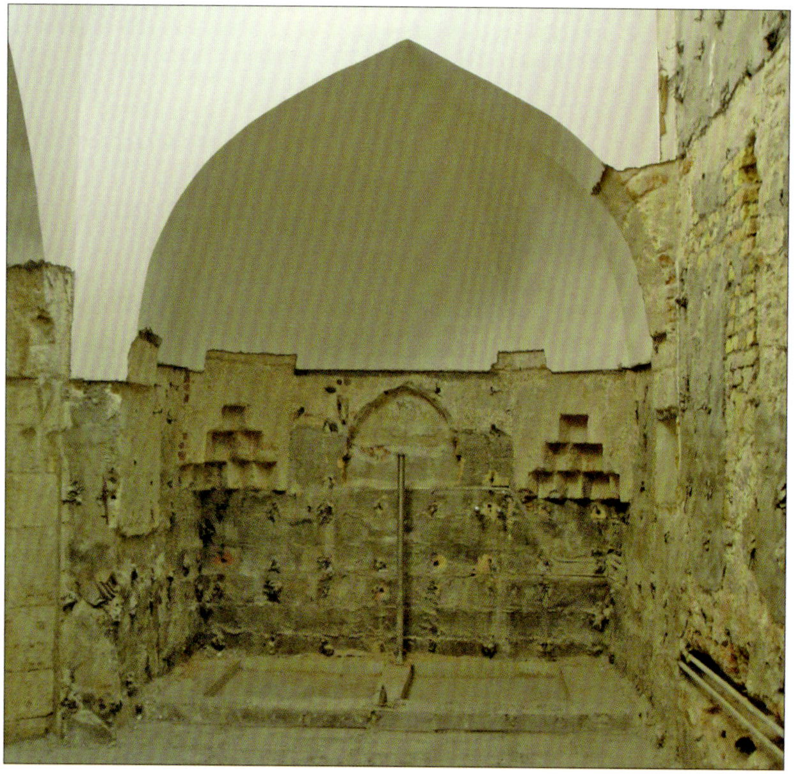

Figure 91. The Császár Baths hot area, *iwans* located on the south side, during excavations

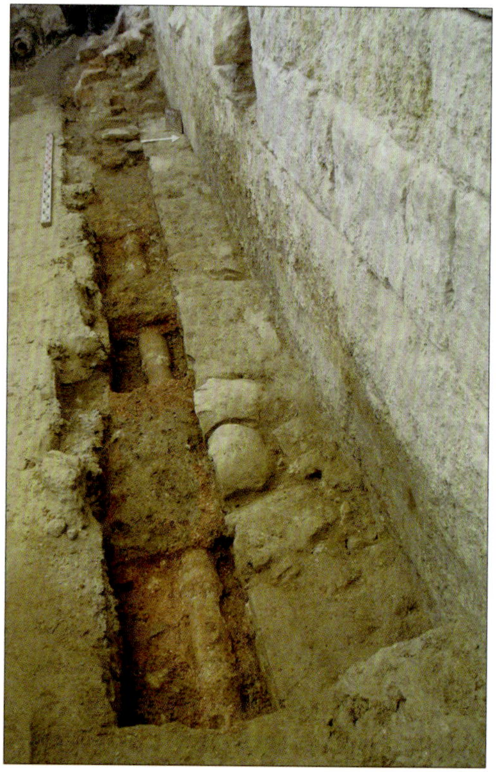

Figure 92. Ottoman era plumbing pipes along the excavated south side of the Császár Baths

The Rác Baths, Buda

Budapest I., Hadnagy utca 8-10.

The Rác Baths are the best-preserved baths in Hungary and include a large section of the entrance hall (*Figure 93*). Archaeological research has exposed the original floor, wall niches, and the source of the water for the baths has also been identified. Thus, it is of this building that the most complete theoretical reconstruction can be made. During their renovation, it was the appearance of the 16th-century baths that was most important; consequently, in Budapest this is where the Ottoman era atmosphere can best be felt (*Figure 94*).

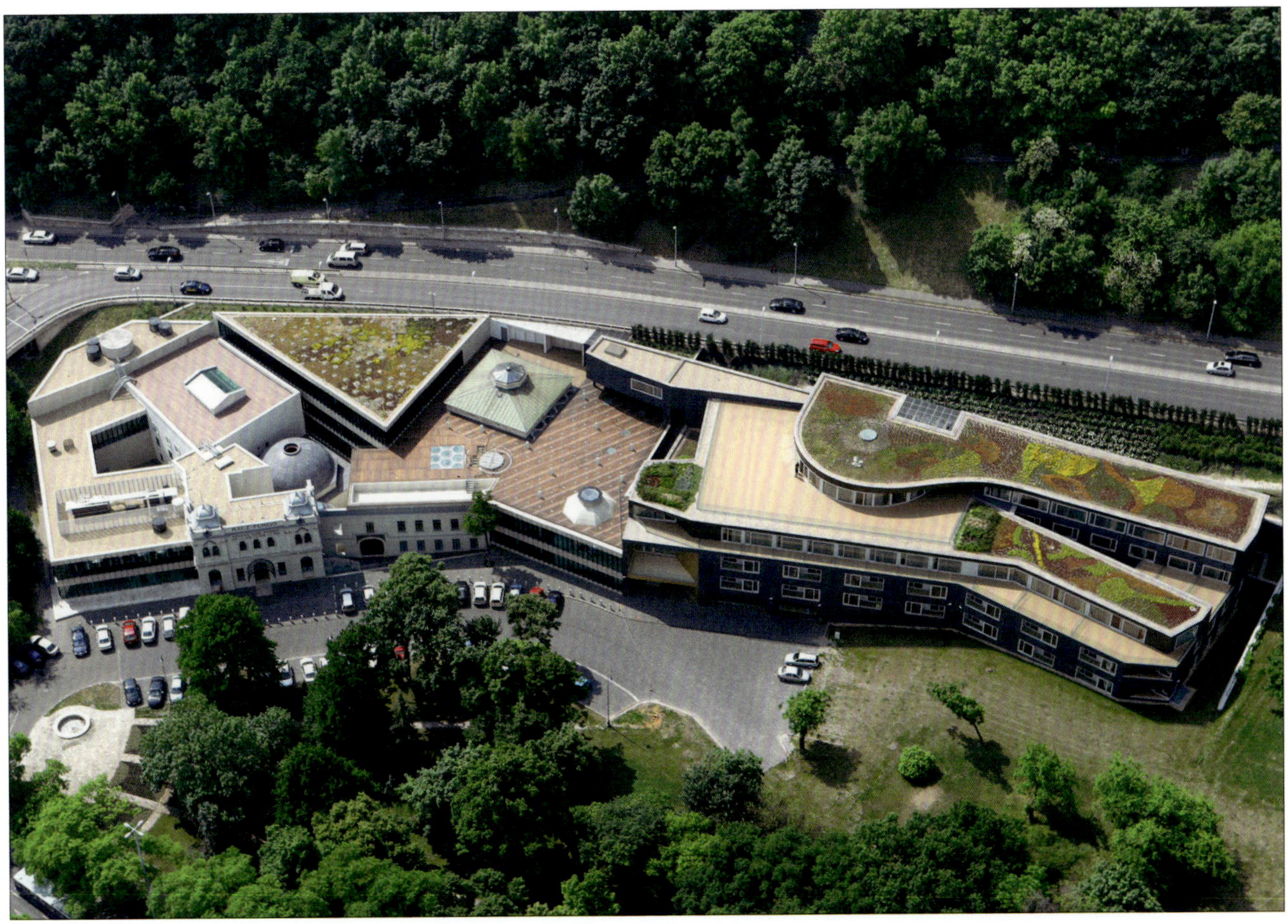

Figure 93. Aerial view of the Rác Baths as they are today. The dome behind the main entrance shows where the Turkish baths stood within the modern building complex

Founder:	unknown
Year of founding:	around 1562
Ottoman era names:	*Debbaghane Ilijasi* (Tabán Baths), *Küchük Ilija* (Little Baths)
Type:	thermal baths
Ground plan type:	star shape (B type) (*Figure 95*)
Director of excavation:	Győző Gerő (1958), Adrienn Papp (2005-2009)
Year of excavation:	1958, 2005-2009
Publications:	Gerő 1980, pp. 96-98; Maráz-Papp 2005; Lászay-Papp 2009

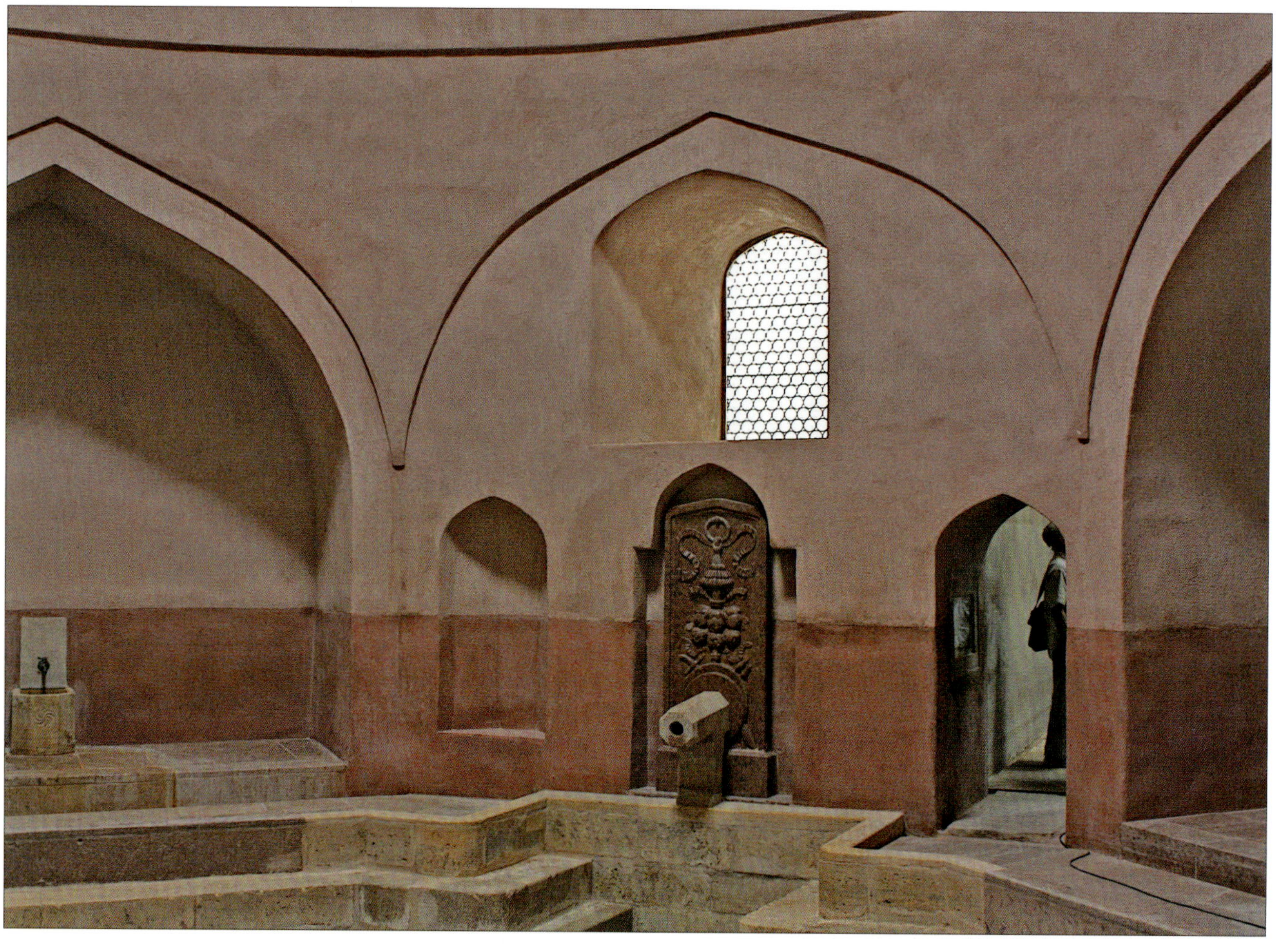

Figure 94. The hot room of the Rác Baths following restoration

HISTORY

These baths were known during the Ottoman era as the Small Baths[113] and as the Taban Baths.[114] The first written record is from 1572 when a traveller, Franciscus Omichius,[115] wrote about two baths at the foot of Gellert Hill that can now be identified as the Rudas and the Rác baths. The records of the Foundation of Sokollu Mustafa Pasha[116] state that it purchased these baths in the tanneries district from the honourable Hassan Mevlana, the one-time *qadi* (judge) of Pest. During the archaeological excavations, wooden posts in good condition were excavated from beneath the Ottoman era walls, dendrochronological study of them revealed 1562 as the likely date of construction.[117] Later, Sokollu Mustafa, Beylerbey of Buda (1566-1578) bought the baths and established the foundation he attached to them.

Two Ottoman era construction periods could be identified during the excavation. In the second of these periods a private bath was added to the baths, and from which well-preserved wooden posts remain. Dendrochronological examination identifies 1588 as the likely date for this extension. In this room several pools were dug. These cannot be dated, but it is possible that they were dug at the same time that the warm rooms were refurbished. Written sources from the Ottoman era commend the baths for their excellent water, which could treat a number of diseases.[118]

According to Marsigli's writings[119] the baths just survived the war of reconquest. Today, the dome from above the entrance hall, parts of the walls, the dome from above the private baths and the walls that supported that are all missing. The dome from the entrance hall must have been destroyed during or shortly after the reoccupation, but the walls survived. De la Vigne's map (1686) only describes a dome over the hot room, not over the entrance hall. It turns out from the writings of Christian travellers that they viewed the baths and the hot room,[120] so it is possible that we should understand Marsigli's phrasing as an indication that the room with the baths did more or less remain.

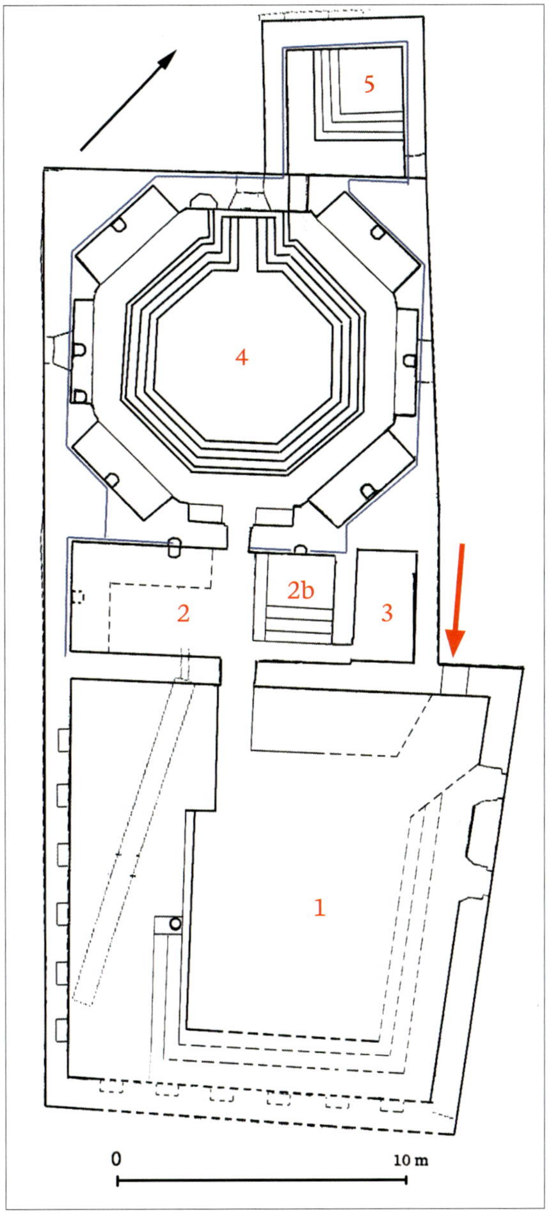

Figure 95. The floorplan of the Rác Baths.
1. Entrance Hall. 2. Warm room.
2b: Pool in the warm room. 3. Toilet.
4. Hot room. 5. Private bath
(the coloured arrow indicates the entrance)

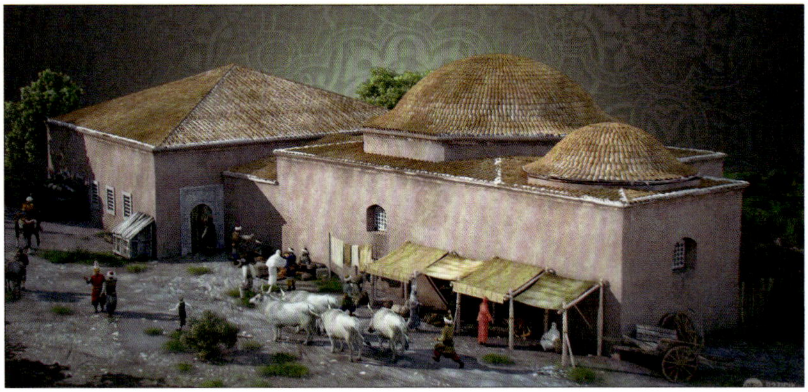

Figure 96. The reconstruction of the Rác Baths

The outline of the baths barely changed until the middle of the 19th century, and the Ottoman era building was visible in the 1721 and 1775 illustrations of the place.[121] The survey sketches also gave the dimensions in Viennese fathoms which, when re-calculated, give the dimensions of the Ottoman era building. However, the transformation of the interior of the building had already begun at that time. The common space in the entrance hall was divided several times, the series of fountains along the wall were shut off, but the building was still used as a bath. During the second half of the nineteenth century, a major spa was built over several phases, with the Ottoman era building at the centre. All the rooms were extant until 1890, but during the transformations then the private baths were demolished. According to the plans made in 1909, the Ottoman era entrance was widened, and the wall between the warm room and the toilets was demolished to widen the entrance to the hot room.[122] On site investigations confirmed that the reconstructions on the plan were indeed completed.

In the 1930s, when the city quarter around the spa was demolished, the spa building was also considered for demolition, but the decision was ultimately rejected. During the Second World War, the bath was heavily damaged and, during the 1960s, the current baths were built from about one third of the 19th-century baths. This third of the building belonged to the Ottoman era building, which suffered relatively minor injury. During the transformation, the south-eastern part of the Ottoman era entrance hall was outside the operating spa building and its walls were dismantled. However, there were changes in the Ottoman era building that do not appear on the floor plans. For example, the floor level was raised–perhaps due to the groundwater level rising in connection with the transformation of the Danube shoreline–but in any case, the Ottoman era floors were not disassembled, rather new layers were added. For this reason, it was necessary to alter the door openings and all the Ottoman era doorways were demolished. The entrance to the private pool alone remain untouched, as shown on a 1873 floor plan[123] although the entrance was walled up, and the private bath was then approached from another direction. In that state, research and renovation began in 2005 by dismantling the 19th-century wing.

DESCRIPTION OF THE BUILDING

During the excavations between 2005-2009, the bath was fully explored: research was carried out on significant surfaces in the building and its surroundings. The bath is located on a northwest-southeast axis between the shore of the 'Devil's Trench' stream and the foot of Gellért Hill. It was in the area built in the Ottoman era, in the city quarter belonging to tanners. On its northeast side there was a square, and a bridge led over the stream to the baths. The bath was 'back to front': the hot room was on the side of the square, while the entrance hall was cut into the foot of the hill. There was a ditch along the southwest side of the spa building (*Figure 96*).

The entrance hall

The walls of the entrance hall are almost all standing, albeit shortened to varying heights, the south-east side having suffered most damage. The room is an irregular rectangle, its location marked out by the spring supplying water to the bath (*Fig. 54*). The natural rock slope is almost 12 meters long, its walls elevated to raise the water level to feed water to the rest of the bath through gravity. The resulting spring outlets were covered and the whole thing arranged along the lines of a raised bench with steps leading to the top. The remaining three walls of the entrance hall are lined with lower benches, more appropriate to Ottoman baths. The steps, the floor and the wall benches were in places excavated in their original locations. The niches of the south-west wall came to light (see *Figure 52*). The south-east wall was probably much the same because behind that wall was the hillside in the Ottoman era, so they couldn't have opened windows. There was no fountain in the middle of the hall, only a small round well, set into the stairway in front of the southwestern wall.

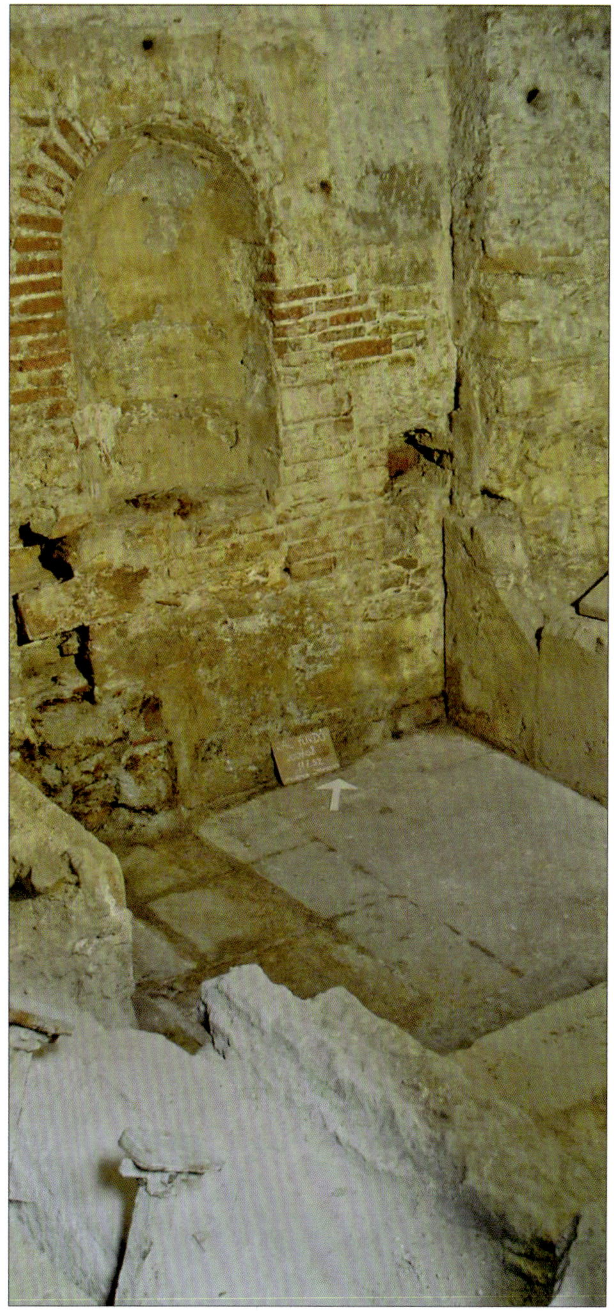

Figure 97. The warm room at the Rác Baths: Ottoman era niche and pool

Given that the entrance hall was not built onto the square next to the building, the entrance is not to be found in the usual place, either. That is generally on the central axis of the building, whereas here it is on the corner of the north-western wall, where the entrance hall wall extends beyond the warm area.

The warm room

The warm room was slightly damaged but did survive. The excavation shows the modern reservoir that was built in the western part of the space is what remains of the Ottoman era water channel. Here, the southeast and northwest wall of the bath are built onto the rock, but not southwest. Thus, it could not have operated as a reservoir during the Ottoman era, but a water channel did pass through it, although we do not know in which direction it went. The room itself was rebuilt in the Ottoman era and the number of fountains and pools was increased. In the first period, there would only have been fountains beneath the niches in the southwestern and northeastern walls. Later, in the eastern part of the room, a swimming pool was set up (*Figure 97*), so the fountains would have been removed.

The walls were plastered here: the remains of pink and red plaster were exposed. There was a window on the south-west sidewall, so skylights can only be found on the eastern side of the barrel vaulting.

The toilet

At the eastern end of the northeastern wall of the warm room, a door opened toward the toilet. From the remains of the door (the door jamb and the beginning of the head), it was possible to construe the one-time door into a lancet arch and stepped decoration. From the toilet only the large channel carried the sewage away from the building. The room is covered with barrel vaulting, above which the layer of Ottoman mortar has been preserved.

The hot room

The hot room was unusually well preserved, even its plasterwork was exposed almost completely intact, only two small modern swimming pools were opened up. On the curb benches next to the walls the the limescale deposits marked the locations of the former fountains, and the red plastering of the walls continued over these little washbasins, that is, they were plastered over.

The slightly protruding rim of the octagonal pool prevented dirty water from running back into the pool. The wall facing the entrance was decorated with three niches, the east of which was converted into a doorway when the private bath was built. The light was provided by three windows. There were no skylights in the dome, but in the centre there was an opening that was enlarged in the 19th century, so the original size is not known. Outside, some fragments of the Ottoman era ledge have survived.

The private bath

In the small square room of the private bath was a small pool in the Ottoman era. This room was built later for the bath, which can be inferred from the design of the doorway, but the transformation of the plumbing system also left informative traces. The hall was covered by a dome, which was demolished by Miklós Ybl; however, fortunately he prepared a survey drawing of the structures before they were dismantled (*Figure 98*). Traces of the dome's structural fitting remained on the northwestern facade of the hot room.

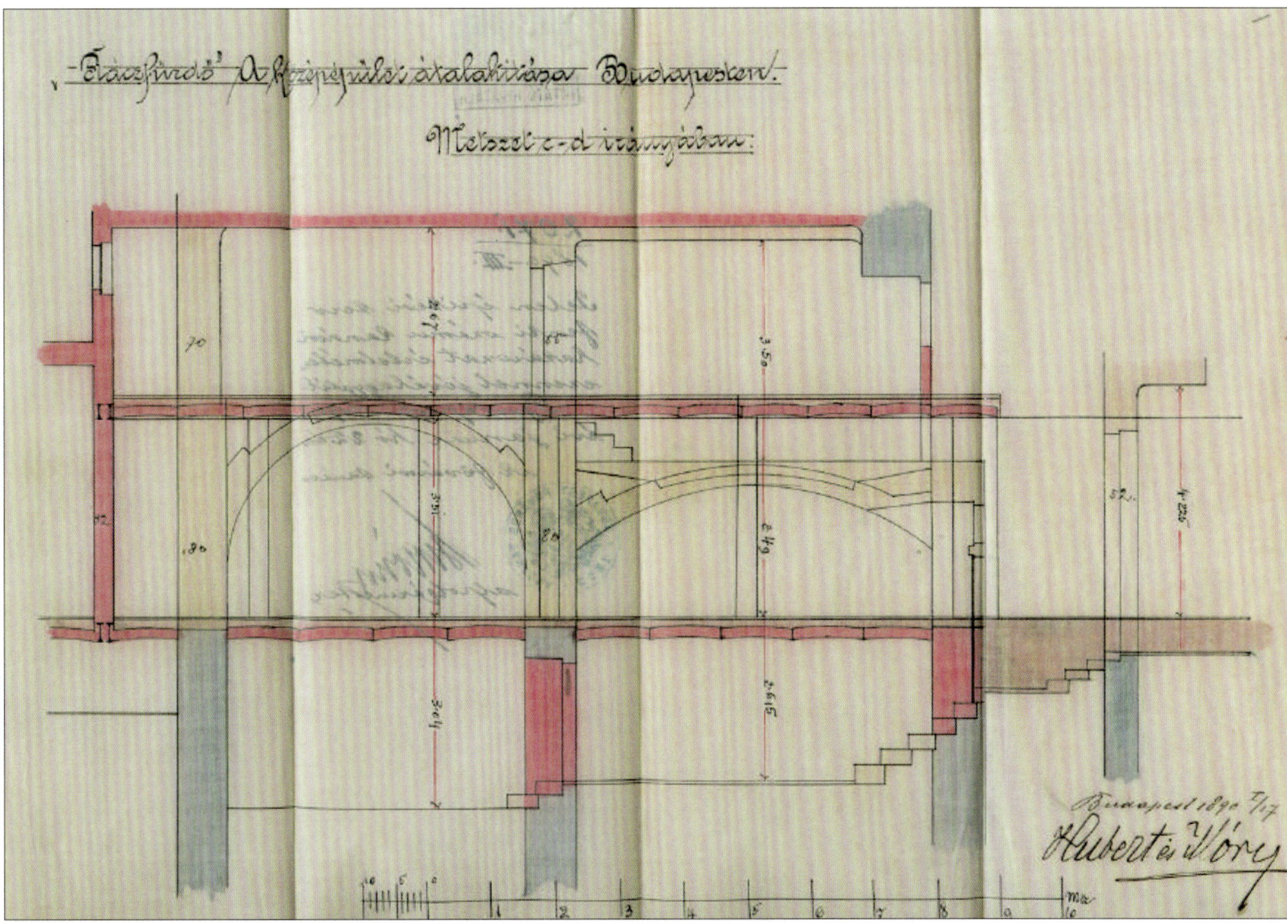

Figure 98. The Rác Baths rebuilding plan from 1890, in which the demolition of the dome to the private bath is represented. Hubert and Móry

The Király Baths, Buda

Budapest II., Fő utca 84.

The Király Baths are of an average size. Their 21st century renovation is still awaited, but in the 1950's it was realised that a significant part of the former baths had survived, even the elevated walls of the entrance hall (*Figure 99*). It is hoped that this renovation will find much preserved in the earth, and that during fresh construction-related research many fascinating details can be revealed.

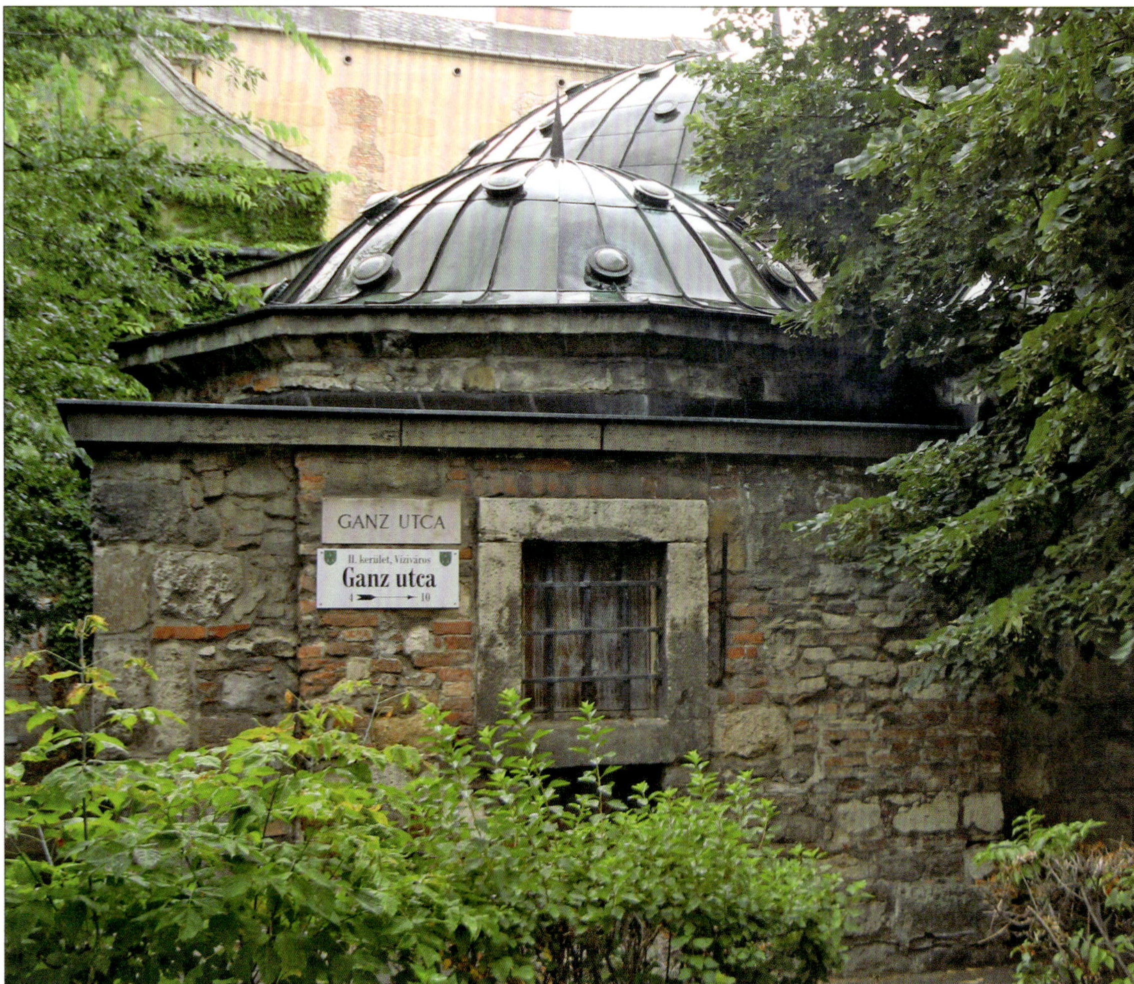

Figure 99. The Király Baths, Buda

Founder:	Sokollu Mustafa Pasha
Year of foundation:	1566–1574
Ottoman era name:	*Horos Kapi Ilijasi* (Cockerel Gate Baths)
Type:	thermal baths
Floor plan type:	star-shaped (B type) (*Figure 100*)
Director of Excavation:	Győző Gerő
Year of Excavation:	1955
Publications:	Gerő 1958; Gerő 1963; Gerő 1980, pp. 90–96

HISTORY

The Király Baths were known in the Ottoman era as the Cockerel Gate Baths (*Horos Kapi Ilijasi*)[124] or as the Baths at the Gate (see Marsigli).[125] The earliest reference is in the foundation book of Sokollu Mustafa, which was written around 1578. In 1572, Franciscus Omichius was perhaps referring to the Király Baths when he wrote: "The third bath, which lies in the direction of Óbuda, was built in the same manner".[126] Since the Császár Baths were only completed in 1574, Omichius could not have seen that, so we can posit 1566–1572 as the probable construction period for the Király Baths.

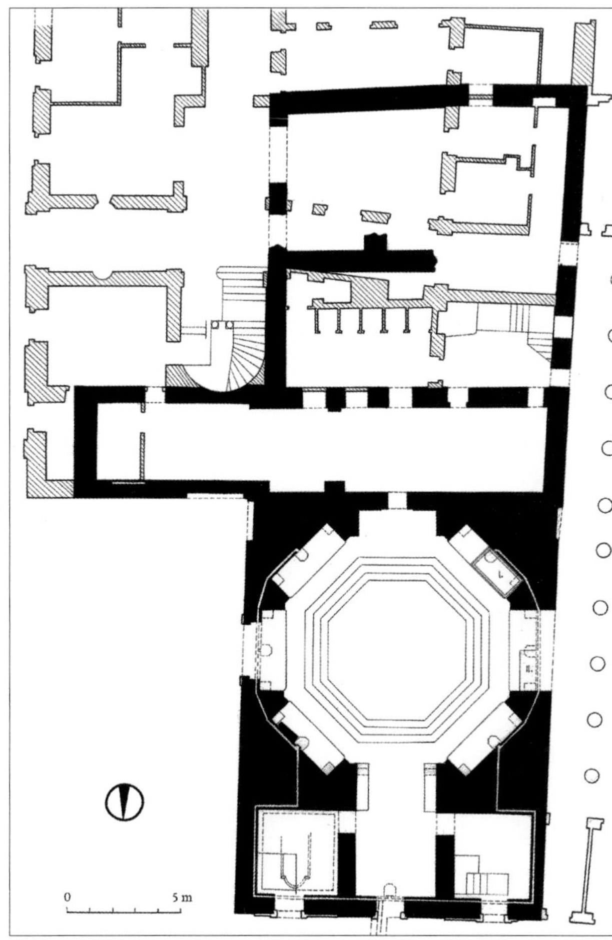

Figure 100. The Király Baths survey plan from 1955

Earlier research[127] revealed that Arslan Pasha, who carried out significant construction in the area, began the building of the Király Baths, which was then completed only by his successor, Sokollu Mustafa Pasha. However, according to recent research, Sokollu Mustafa Pasha (1566–1578) clearly also raised this bath.[128] The last renovation of the building and the related research took place in 1954–1959. At that time, several Ottoman era construction periods were not separated,[129] but traces of renovations were identified: the modifications to the roof and the replacement of the roof tiles was dated to the 17th century.[130]

The year of Edward Brown's visit, the spa burnt down in the great fire of Buda in 1669, but was then refurbished and used once more.[131] From the war of reconquest, however, it

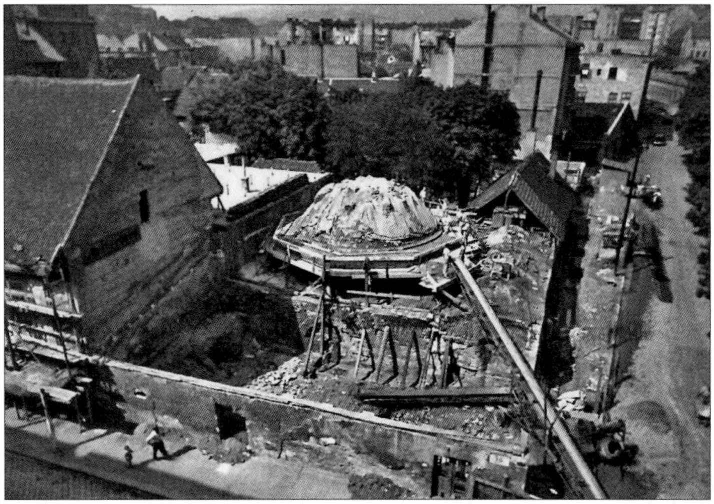

Figure 101. Research on the Király Baths in 1954-1959

survived intact,[132] although it is not out of the question that the entrance hall was damaged then. On March 3, 1687, the spa had a new owner. In the 18th and 19th centuries, major reconstruction took place, when it was renovated and restructured according to the needs of the day. In the 18th century, the Ottoman building and the area surrounding it were built over, and in the 19th century the baths were enlarged with a grand classicist building.[133] The Ottoman era building, including the domes, remained intact through the Second World War. During the renovation of 1954-1959, archaeological research into the baths was carried out, during which the Ottoman era parts were identified and

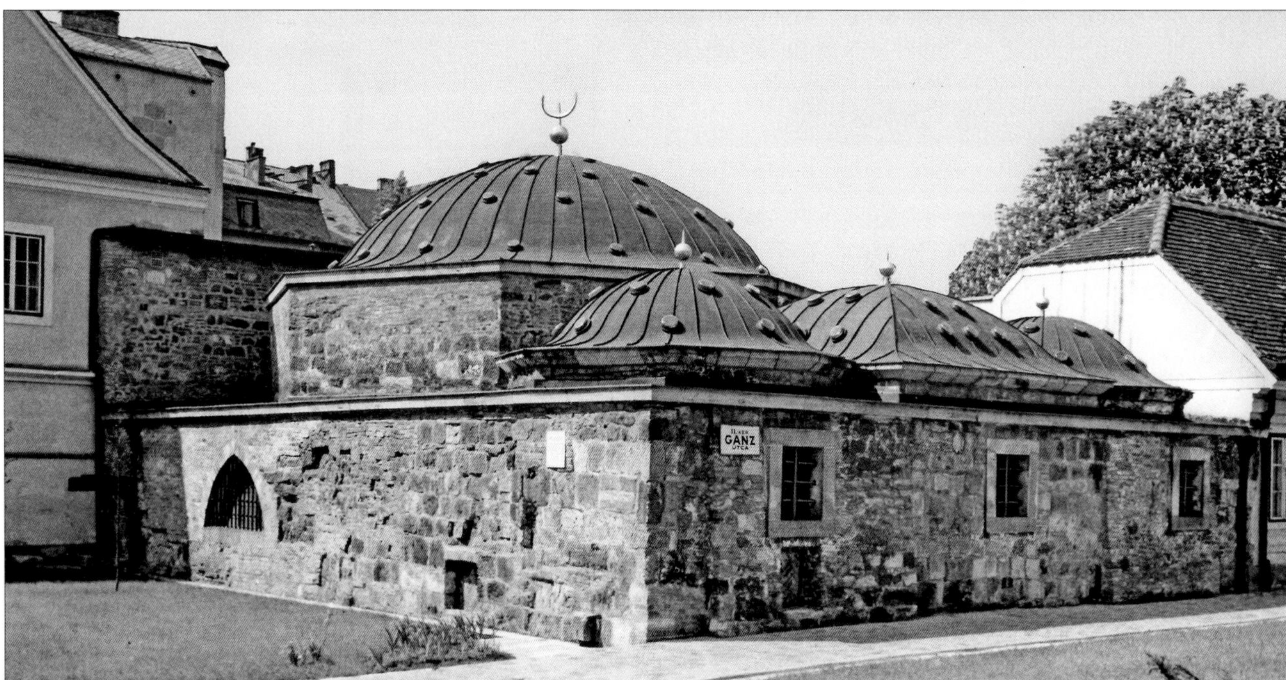

Figure 102. The Király Baths in the 1960s, following refurbishment

the domes were liberated (*Figure 101*). The research was conducted by Győző Gerő. The renovation created the present appearance of the spa (*Figure 102*). Since then, there has been no major refurbishment or research.

DESCRIPTION OF THE BUILDING

Győző Gerő carried out the research into the building in 1955, in connection with its reconstruction. He identified the Ottoman era parts among the buildings from various periods and searched for some detail of the Ottoman building on a small area. The baths stood beside one of the entry points to the city, the Cockerel Gate, on the North-South main road. The baths are interesting because the thermal water is piped to it from the group of springs 700 meters north of the baths. It was the only thermal baths located within the Ottoman city fortifications.

The entrance hall

In the course of his research, Győző Gerő found that the walls of the Ottoman era entrance hall are of varying height but can be found in today's building. The western wall of the bath reaches the first floor of today's building, its high-placed window is still visible (*Figure 103*). On the other sides, only the base walls are extant. No original flooring or wells were exposed.

The warm area

Reconstruction of the warm room raises many questions. The floor plan published by Győző Gerő shows a long room that extends beyond the hot room and the entrance hall. This is a rather strange solution and it differs from that generally used in the era concerned. It is likely that it was divided into several parts, but we do not know exactly how.

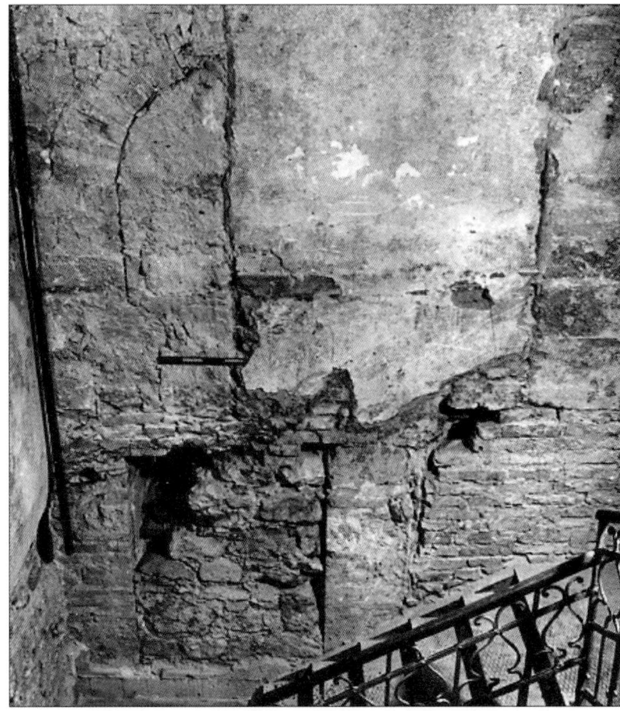

Figure 103. Ottoman era window uncovered during restoration work at the Király Baths

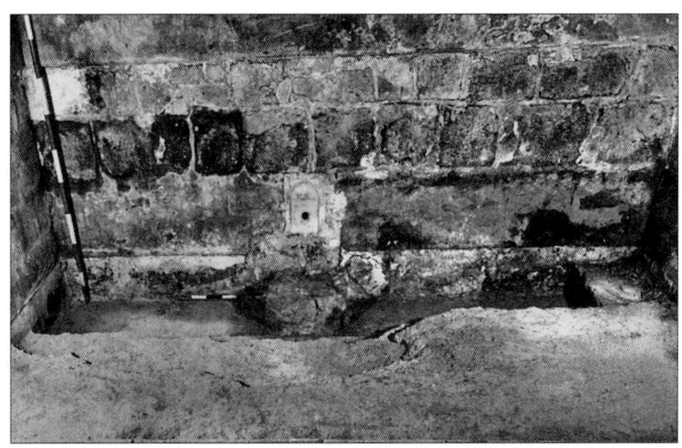

Figure 104. The original flooring and wall fountain of the Ottoman era hot room at the Király Baths

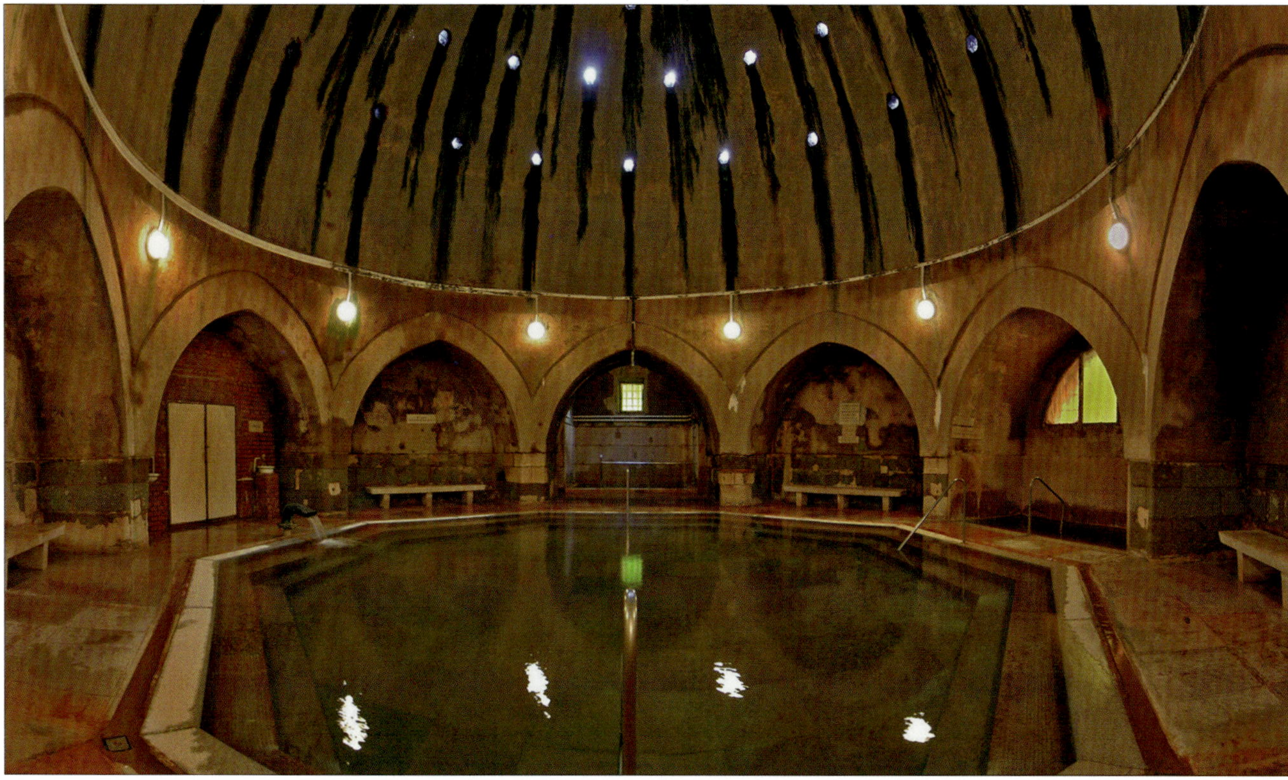

Figure 105. The hot room at the Király Baths as it is today

The hot room

The original stone flooring, the wash basins standing on them, the fronts of the fountains, and some of the original steps into the pool were exposed during the research. From these things we may suppose that there were benches in the large niches in the walls upon which the stone basins were placed. The significance of the fountain found here is that the remains of the basin and its front were preserved in this place alone (*Figure 104–105*).

The private baths

There are three rooms connected to the hot room, among which the two furthest were certainly private baths. However, the precise design of these can not be explored because of the pools constructed in the modern era. In the middle room there was a fountain. Győző Gerő assumed that the bath was supplied with water from this.

The 18th-century roof to the baths was dismantled during the refurbishment work of the 1960s, bringing the Ottoman era domes came to light once more.

Bath ruins open to visitors

Eger: The Valide Sultan Baths

Eger, Tinódi Sebestyén tér 3. (Dózsa György tér 1., later Dobó István utca 7.)

Built beside the gates of Eger Castle, the ruins of the former Valide Sultan Baths can once again be seen after a long period of neglect (*Figure 106*). Once archaeological research was complete, the ruins had to wait for decades to be decently presented, and as a consequence some parts have deteriorated even further. As a result of restoration work completed in 2013, the remains of this building can now be visited once more. In one half of the building the walls remain to the height of the arches, while the other half has been demolished to floor level during modern construction work. The size of the entire building, however, gives a clear sense of the character of each of the rooms as one walks around it.

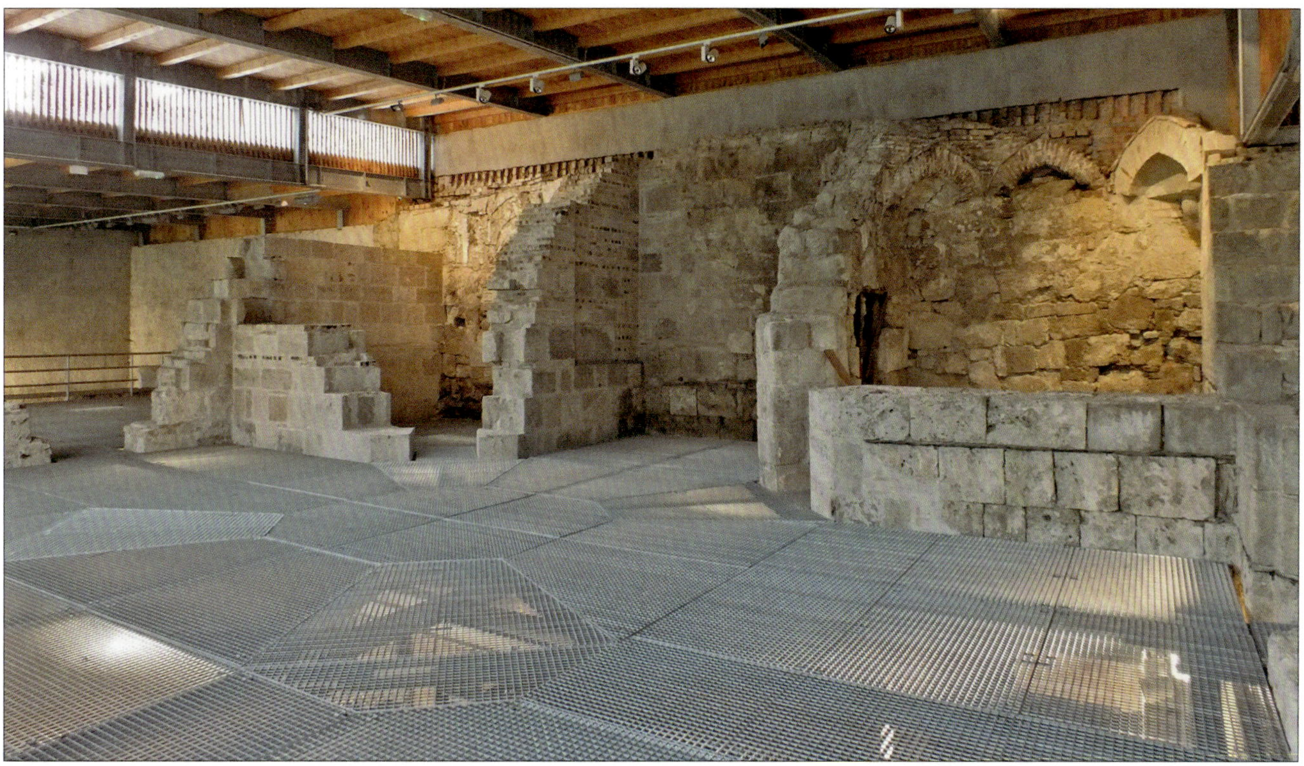

Figure 106. The ruins of the Valide Sultan Baths in Eger today

Founder:	unknown
Constructed:	around 1600
Ottoman era name:	*Valide Sultan Hamami* (Baths of the sultan's mother)
Type:	steam baths
Floorplan type:	cross-shaped (A type) (*Figure 107*)
Director of excavation:	Győző Gerő
Year of excavation:	1958, 1962, 1984–1988
Publications:	Gerő 1980, pp. 106–109, Gerő 1972, pp. 276–280

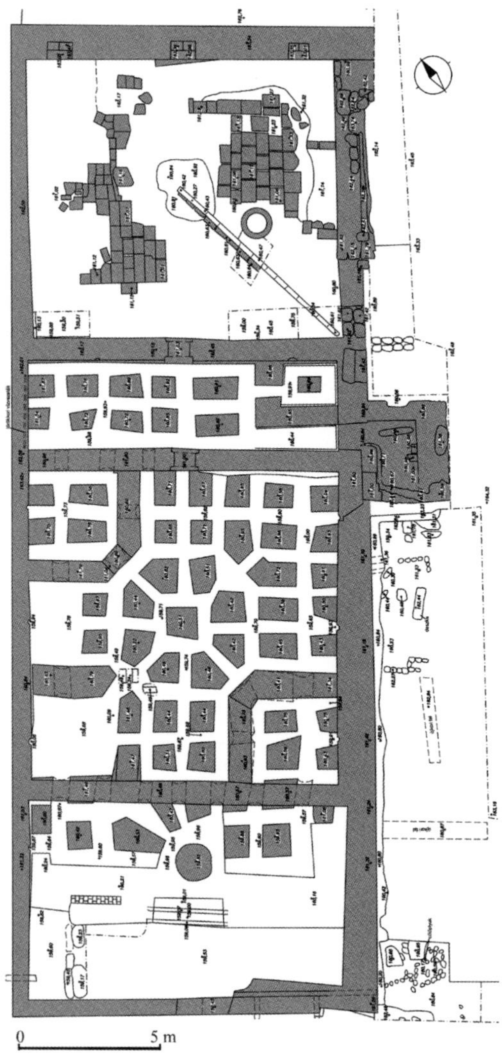

HISTORY

We know next to nothing about the history of these baths. Neither the precise date of completion nor the original name are known. When the town was retaken, the building, as with other steam baths, was used, but no longer as baths. Despite that, sources from the mid 18th century also refer to them as Turkish baths. Its last room was demolished in 1856, and the entire baths were uncovered in the excavations lead by Győző Gerő.

DESCRIPTION OF THE BUILDING

Extending northeast to southwest, the baths stood close to the castle gates. The northwestern wall remains standing to the height of the arches, while the rest has been raised to the foundations. Small areas of its pink and red plaster can still be seen.

The entrance hall

The stone flags of the entrance hall and the stone benches that lined the walls remain, the location of the fountain at the centre is also clearly visible, too. The water mains carried the water from the southern corner of the room to the fountain. Exposed breastwork indicates the location of the niches in the extant walls. The entrance to the baths was not in the axis of the room, but rather in its southeastern corner. The entrance to the warm room was in the middle of the southwestern wall.

Figure 107. Floorplan to the ruins of the Valide Sultan Baths in Eger, 1989

The warm rooms

The rectangular room is divided into two parts: from the eastern corner a narrow corridor leads alongside a smaller seperated area to the toilet. Across most of the room, only the support columns of the floor heating system are visible, but in the western corner only we find the remains of the stone flags from Ottoman era. Impressions can be found in the pink plasterwork. In the south western wall some fragments of the water pipes are visible. Set on the stone wallbench in the larger room was a wall fountain, and it seems highly likely that there was also one in the smaller room, although the walls have deteriorated so much that the level of the water pipes is not discernable.

The toilet

The function of the small square room attached to the outside of the southeastern wall is evident in the broad drain leading out of the building.

The hot room

The former decorative design of the baths can only be reconstructed on the basis of the elevated parts of the western wall. Regrettably, due to neglect in the decades following the initial research, the walls have been deteriorating since the excavations. The arrangement of the room follows the classical conventions: the private baths in the four corners are divided into almost equal sizes that open from the central area–the most common arrangement for this floorplan type. At the centre of the room, the location of a probably octagonal naval stone is indicated by the support columns from the underfloor-heating system (*Figure 108*). Between the private baths wall fountains ran from niches.

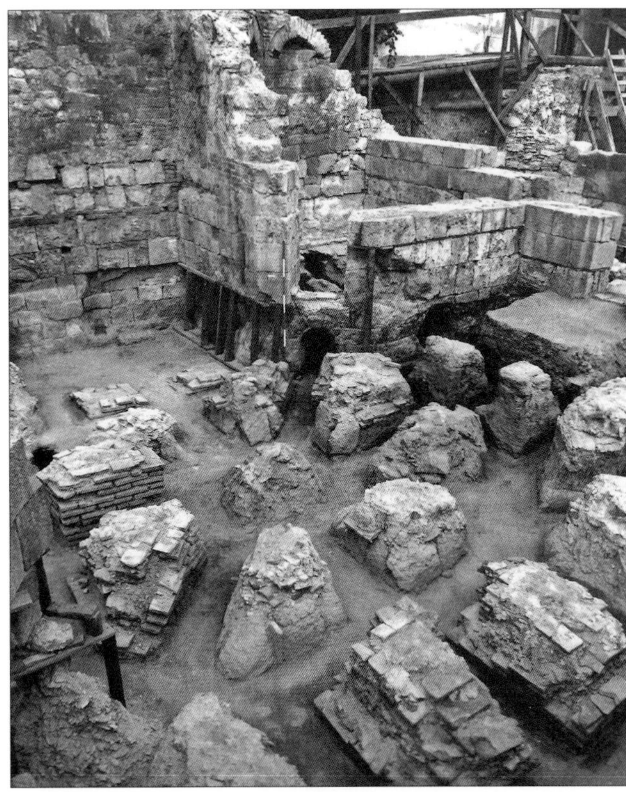

Figure 108. The hot room of the Valide Sultan Baths during its excavation (1980s)

The private baths

The individual baths were placed one in each corner and covered by a cupola, the dome of which was supported by spandrels from the corners. The walls were decorated with niches, and fountains were placed on the main supporting walls in which water pipes could be sited. Evliya Chelebi counted six *halvets*,[134] but we don't know how he came to that figure because if they had also led here then there would have been seven or eight, and if he counted the warm small room, then there would have been five.

The boiler room

The area described by the walls is divided into two areas. The cistern was situated over the underfloor-heating support pillars, and the southern part was used as a woodstore from whence the furnace was fed that warmed the water.

Székesfehérvár: double baths (Güzelje Rüstem Pasha Baths?)

Székesfehérvár, Jókai utca 2. (Ottoman courtyard)

The ruins of Ottoman era double baths in Szekesfehervar town centre are a sad example of how easily ruins degenerate when left without a cover in open ground. The scattered stones and bricks and the covering of weeds are a depressing sight (*Figure 109*). The ruins are obscured particularly well by the building standing beside them, which continues on from the bath building. The area serves as an atmospheric transit zone, but does not really allow us a sense of the buildings themselves. The local environment has been put in some sort of order, but the ruins of the building require protection, otherwise they will just continue to degenerate unstopably. The remaining ruins in their current form are not enough to describe the Turkish baths to those who are not experts in the subject.

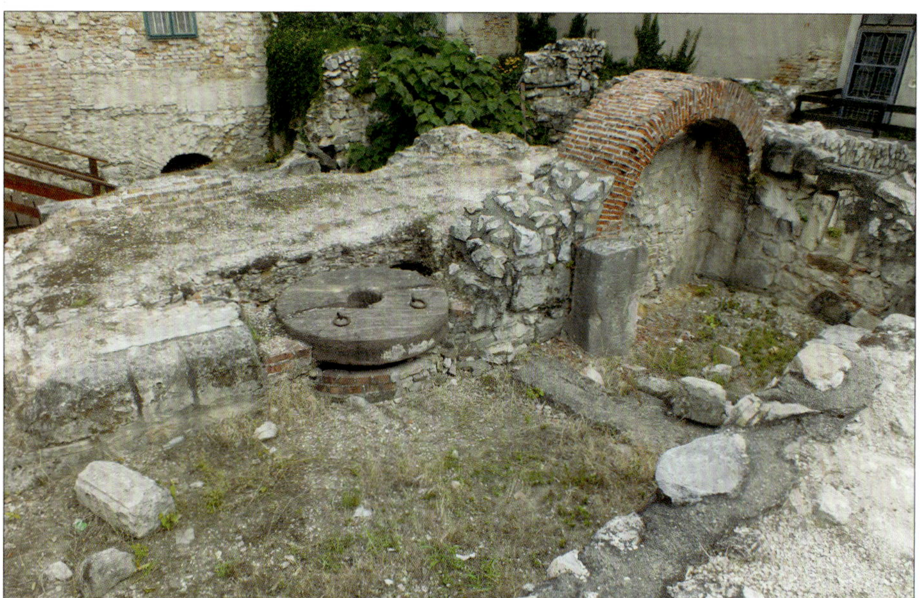

Figure 109. The remains of the double baths in Székesfehérvár as they are today

Founder:	Güzelje Rüstem Pasha or Sokollu Mustafa Pasha
Completed:	prior to 1578
Ottoman era name:	unknown
Type:	steam baths, double baths
Groundplan type:	the male part is a star-shaped (B type); the women's part a centrally-domed central E type (*Figure 110*)
Directors of excavation:	Győző Gerő, Gyula Siklósi
Excavation year:	Gerő 1960?, Siklósi 1987-1988, 1991
Publications:	Gerő 1980, pp. 109-110; Siklósi 1988; Siklósi 1989a; Siklósi 1989b; Siklósi 1990; Siklósi 2013

DESCRIPTION OF THE BUILDING

The baths are close to the city wall beside the road leading to the main square. The hot rooms, private baths and boiler room are all known. We can assume that the larger, southern part was used by men, and that the smaller more modest northern part was used by women.

The male baths

The excavations exposed a six-sided open room was exposed niches in the walls. With this type of baths it is more usual to have niches on eight sides, but the solution in Székesfehérvár can be seen elsewhere in a number of Ottoman baths.[135] One interesting feature of the room is that one of the niches still has a stalectite decoration in situ. This suggests that the niches were covered by cloister vault and that they supported the central dome. Through the western niche, two adjacent baths were discovered that were filled from pipes in the western wall (*Figure 111*).

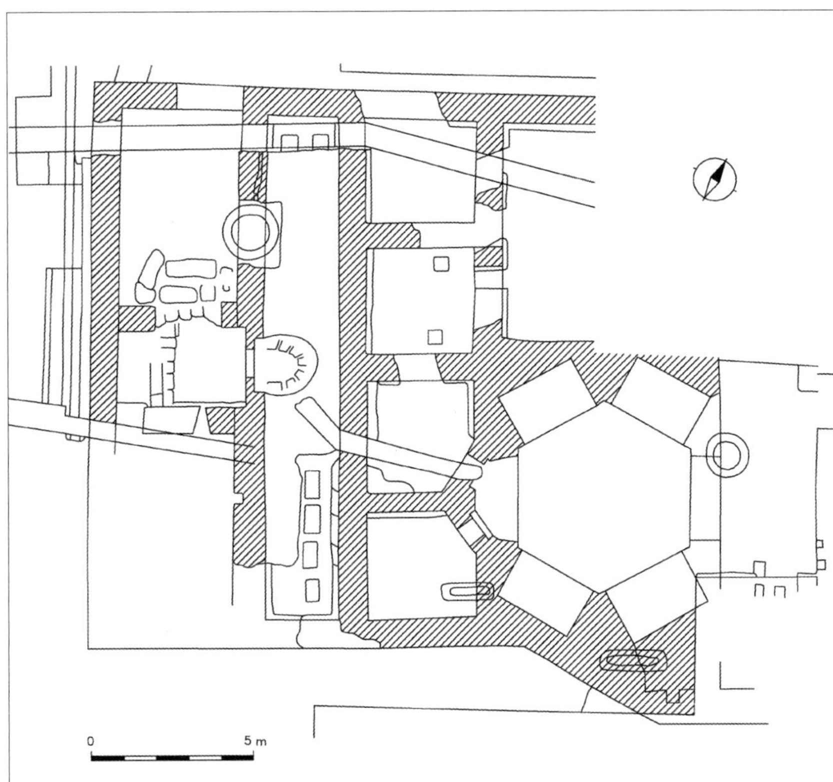

Figure 110. The ground plan of the double baths in Székesfehérvár

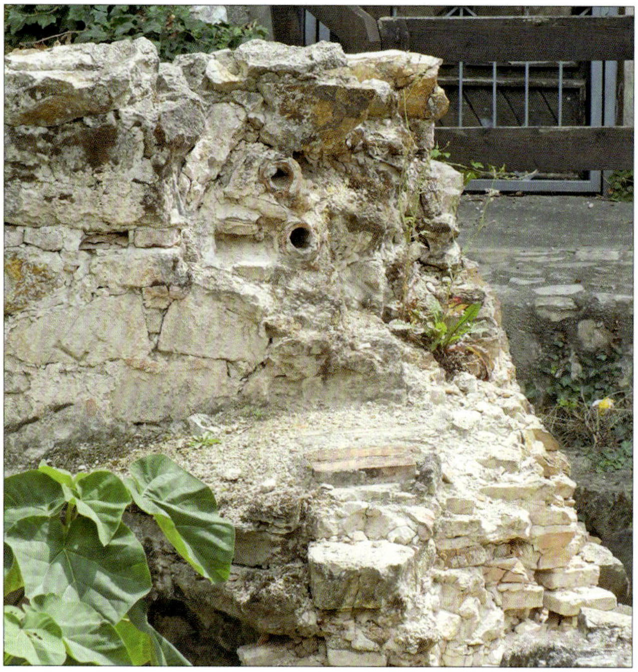

Figure 111. The water pipes visible in the wall of the double baths at Székesfehérvár

The women's baths

Only a fragment of the women's hot room came to light. The width of the building presumably equalled the width of the private baths. Two private baths joined the hot bath area and their wall fountains were situated in the western walls according to the excavating archeologists.

Boiler room, cistern

The boiler room building and the cistern were excavated and stretched across the width of both the male and female parts. The underfloor-heating piller system and parts of the floor can be seen beneath the cistern.

Next to nothing is known of the entrance hall to the baths and the warm areas. Gyula Siklósi's reconstruction shows both parts of the baths reached the street with the entrance hall to the woman's part being rectangular. It could be easily imagined that the entrance hall to the women's part was placed slightly further back. The hot room in the women's was necessarily the same width as the private baths togeter. The groundplans of the entrance halls were more or less square and during this period they did not tend to extend beyond the line of the building. In which case the walls of the women's bath lay approximately four metres from the street. A rectangular entrance hall or one protruding from the side of the building is not out of the question either. Although the issue can only be satisfactorily resolved with further excavations.

Pécs: The Memi Pasha Baths

Pécs, Ferencesek utcája 64.

The Memi Pasha Baths, converted from the buildings of a mediaeval Franciscan Church, were still standing at the end of the 19th century beside the mosque, close to the Sziget Gate on the western mediaeval city walls of Pécs. The condition of the baths has been much better preserved than in Székesfehérvár (*Figure 112*). One reason for this was that during excavation the walls were exposed in a ruinous condition, and in an effort to conserve them they were rebuilt. In the decades that have passed since then, this ruin has suffered and only part of the once completely reconstructed well now stands. However, the size of the buildings and the character of the rooms can be sensed clearly.

Founder:	Memi Pasha
Year of founding:	unknown
Ottoman era name:	*Memi Pasha Hamami* (Memi Pasha Baths)
Type:	steam baths
Groundplan type:	the male part had an E-type central dome, but the female part cannot be determined (*Figure 113*)
Director of excavation:	Győző Gerő
Year of excavation:	1977
Publications:	Gerő 1987

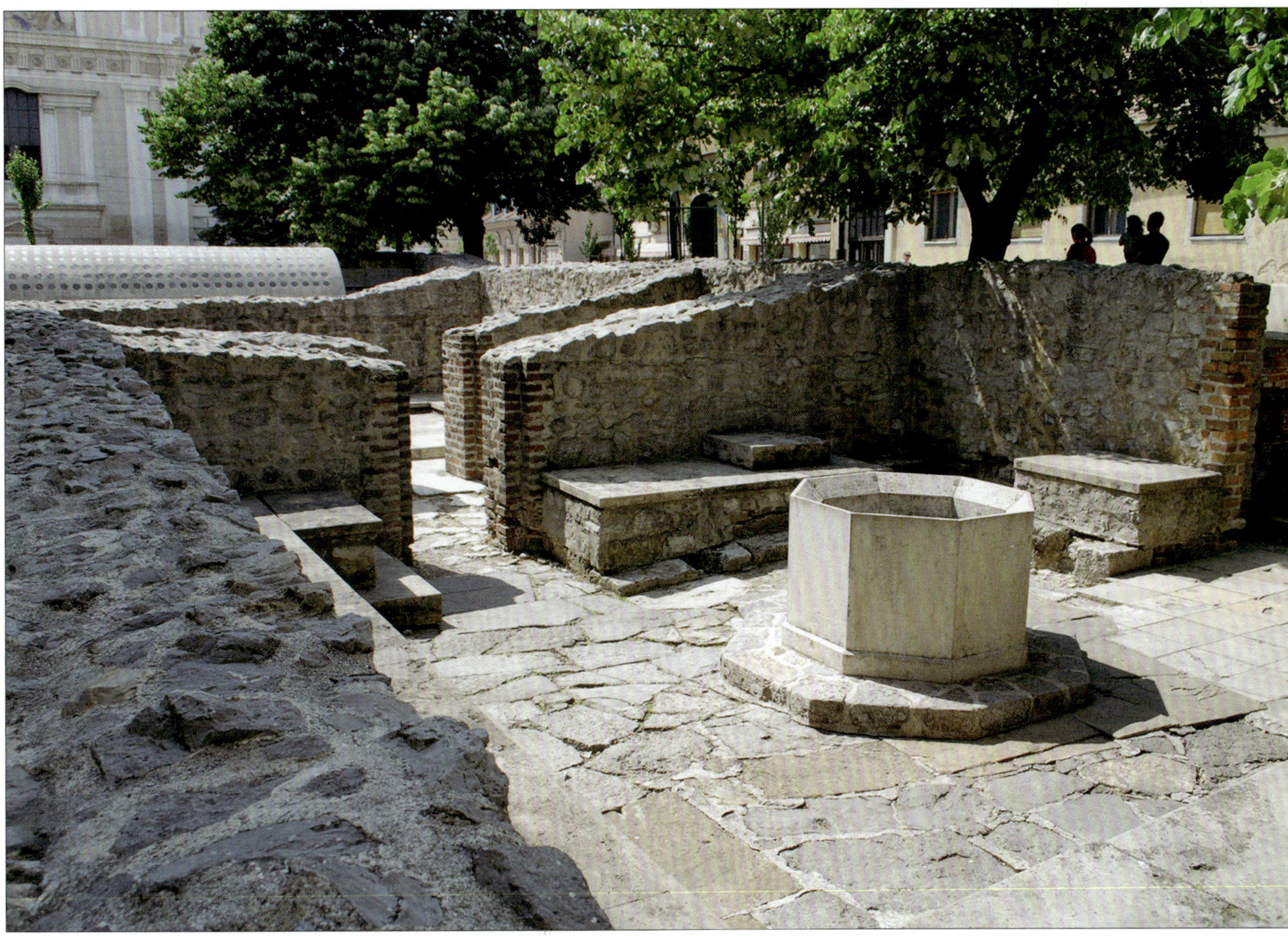

Figure 112. The ruins of the Memi Pasha Baths in Pécs as they are today

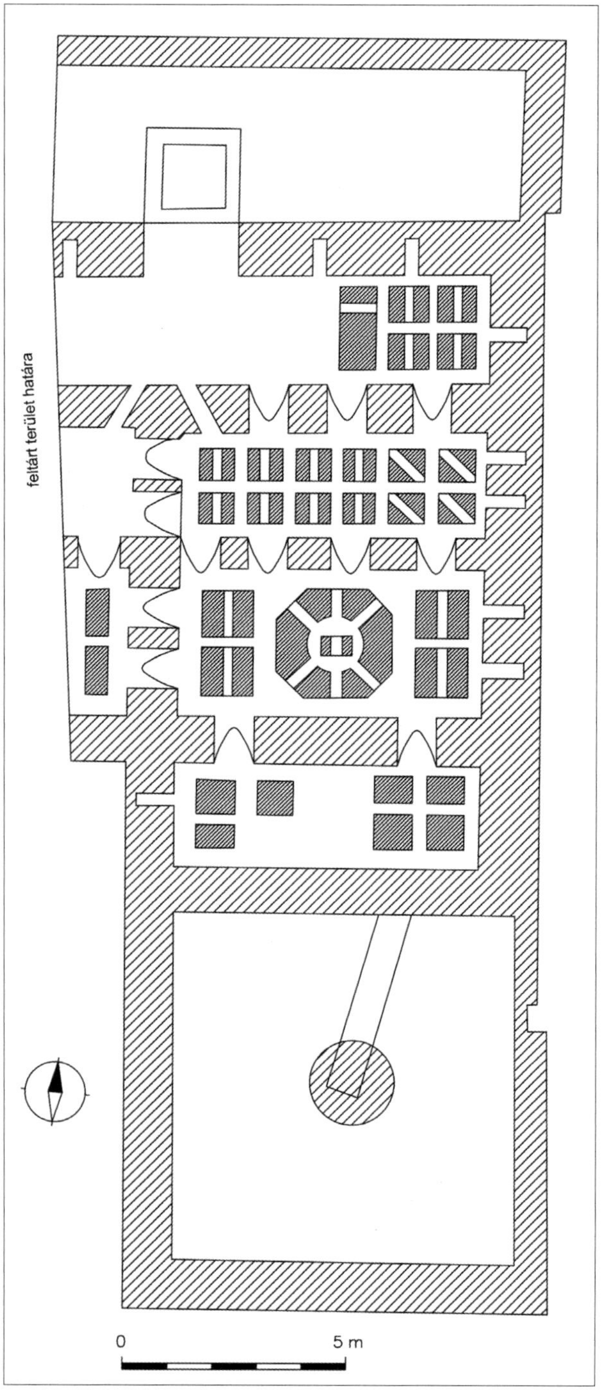

Figure 113. The floorplan of the Memi Pasha Baths

DESCRIPTION OF THE BUILDING

Only one half of the double baths was raised, but that part in its entirety. The entrance hall was exposed, its floor and central fountain. Of the remaining rooms only the walls above floor level and the supporting pillars from the underfloor heating system appeared. These provided an opportunity to clarify the groundplan, the form of the naval stone is always marked out by its supports for presumably structural reasons. The fallen dividing walls are also some distance from the underfloor-heating supports. All of which makes likely a layout at odds with the current reconstruction, that is of the E-type, double private baths. The excavation drawings and photographs clearly show that at the centre of the square area there was a dividing wall on the east side of which the naval stone was located, now marked out by the octagonal arrangement of support pillars. The dividing wall between the private baths cannot now be identified, but given that the drawing and the photograph do not entirely match, the central line of pillars could well have been the remains of the demolished wall. For that there is no clear answer as to why the dividing walls should have decayed more completely than the others, whether it was as a result of Ottoman, or Modern Age modification, or for some other unknown reason.

The cistern and the boiler room were uncovered west of the hot room, and the stumps of the wall that carried on into the southern part double baths.

Bath ruins with limited access

Buda: Beylerbey's Palace private baths

Budapest I., Színház utca 5-9.

The private baths of the Beylerbeys of Buda were in the castle at Buda. The remains of the former Carmelite Monastery (later the Castle Theatre) can be found in the cellar (*Figures 114–115*), much visited by experts and archaeologists in the long period following the excavations, but not open to the general public. Hidden among the cables and pipes, you can get close to the walls, and enter the hot room through the opening to the boiler room or by climbing over the cistern. The Prime Minister's Office plans to take possession of the building, thus it awaits its presentation. It is worth taking into public ownership given the remarkable nature of the ruins, and as the only known complete private bath in the country. In the small, well-defined ruin, all the rooms of the bath, even the boiler room are viewable.

Founder:	unknown
Year of founding:	circa 1600
Ottoman era name:	unknown
Type:	steam baths
Groundplan type:	single dome (H type) (*Figure 116*)
Director of excavation:	Győző Gerő
Year of excavation:	1955, 1966
Publications:	Gerő 1968; Gerő 1980, 112–115; Gerő 1999; Papp 2013

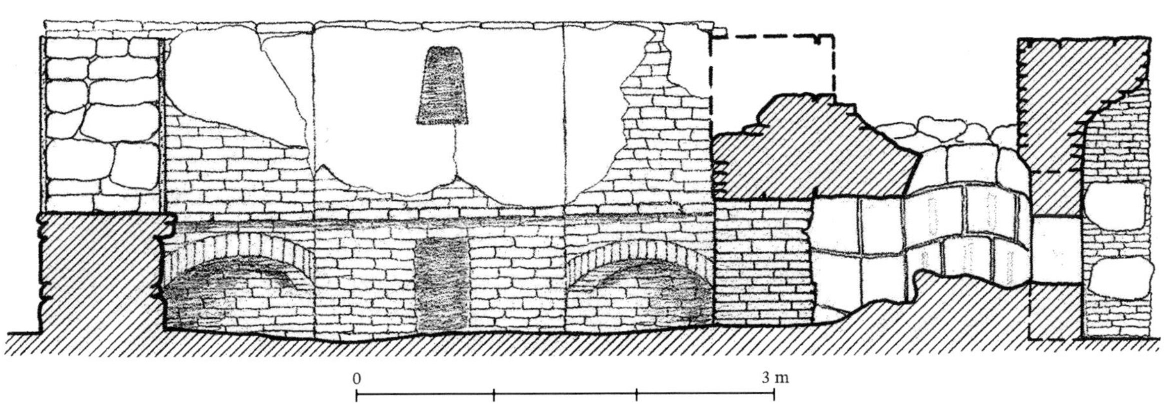

Figure 114. Excavation drawings of the private baths of the Beylerbey's Palace in Buda from 1955

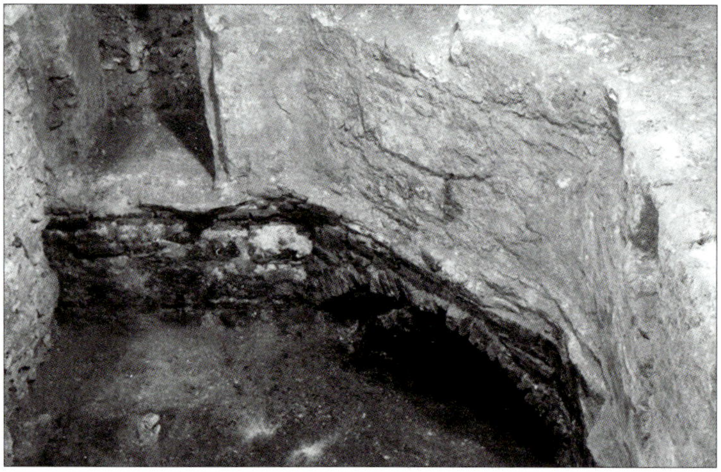

Figure 115. The remains of the hot room of the private baths of the Beylerbey's Palace in Buda, 1966

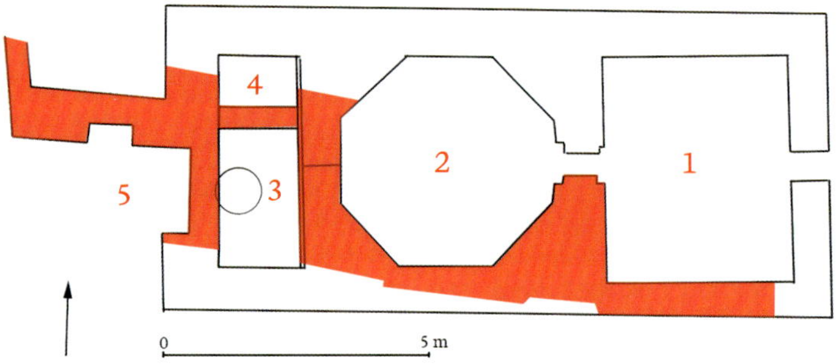

Figure 116. The excavation drawing of the private baths of the reconstructed Beylerbey's Palace in Buda, the excavated parts are highlighted. 1. Warm room. 2. Hot room. 3. Hot water cistern. 4. Cold water cistern. 5. Heating room

HISTORY

We know nothing of the sixteenth-century palace—or palaces—of the Beylerbey of Buda, so it is not out of the question that it or they included a private bath. It is made likely on the one hand by the Ottoman tradition of attaching baths to palaces; and on the other hand that Reinhold Lubenau, the Emperor's ambassador from Königsberg wrote in 1587 that the Beylerbey of Buda had both bath and garden.[136] The lack of richer written sources is not decisive, since the 17th-century private baths are mentioned only by Evliya Chelebi and by Luigi Ferdinando Marsigli, a scientist from Italy.[137] All this suggests that the Western ambassadors were not aware of the baths of the Pasha in the 17th century—so it was likely thus in the 16th century.

The most detailed description of the Beylerbey's palace was made by Evliya Chelebi,[138] and the Western ambassadors only saw and mentioned the reception hall (*Figure 117*). The building of the palace by Khodja Musa Pasha (1631-1634, 1637-1638, 1640-1644) was linked to the possibility of drawing water from the Danube into the Castle. We know that the only fountain to which water was run from the Danube stood beside the Beylerbey of Buda's palace.[139] Its location cannot be accidental: the water-drawing facility would not only have supplied this one fountain with water, but other parts of the palace as well, such as the baths.

The building was either built when the palace was created or during the later expansion of the building; the currently available archaeological data is insufficient to decide with any certainty. Following the war of reconquest, during the building of the new Carmelite monastery, the building was partially demolished and the rubble from the walls was used as hard core to establish the new floor level of the palace. The area remained that way until the post-Second World War restoration work began and the excavations when, within the framework of the research into the Palace of Buda between 1958 and 1968, Győző Gerő discovered the remains of the baths.

DESCRIPTION OF THE BUILDING

The baths were in a separate building of the palace, which was located in the private part of the palace. It was north of the large courtyard and opened from a smaller courtyard. The two rooms of the baths were completely excavated in 1966 along with the boiler room.

The entrance hall

In the case of private pools, the functions of the entrance hall and the warm area can be covered by the same room. This can be seen here: one of the baths is in a small rectangular room underneath which the underfloor heating system does not go. No water pipes have been found in what remains of the walls. The entrance supposedly opened from the east because its northern side was so very close to the border of the palace, and on its southern side there was a contiguous wall, which certainly did not have a door.

The hot room

On its outer side it forms a square, the inner walls, however, form an octagon. The columns from the underfloor heating system are known, and the wall identifies the level of the former floor. The walls were covered with pink plaster. Research identified water pipes in the western wall where water was brought across from the neighboring cistern, and there probably would have been a fountain here also. There were no wells on the southern side and its demolition means we do not know about the north side.

Due to the size of the building, the stone wall benches and the naval stone wouldn't fit into the space together at the same time. The columns of the underfloor heating system do not draw the naval stone's outline, and the line of the demolished floor on the wall appears uniform. For this reason, the interior layout of the room is unclear.

The boiler room

The western side of the baths close with the cisterns and the heating room. Two tanks can be identified, underneath one is the furnace with its opening which was covered by a copper bowl which held the boiling water. Under the other tank there is nothing similar, so it was probably a cold water tank. The fire under the hot water tank could be fed from the west side. One particularly interesting feature is that that the protective wall around the heating house was visible.

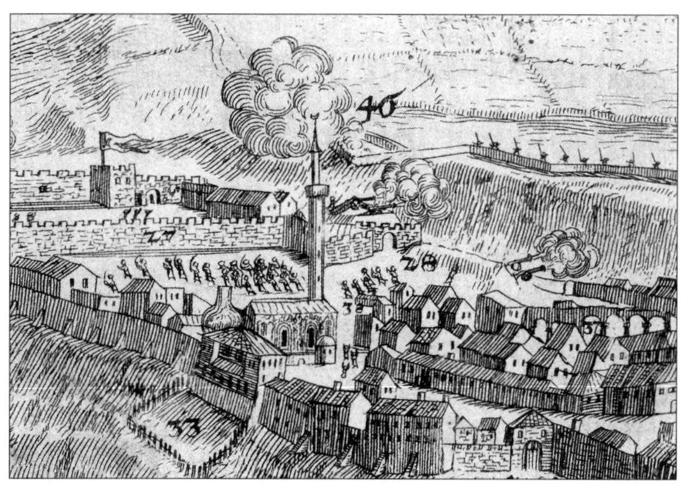

Figure 117. An engraving of the 1686 siege of Buda by Domenico Fontana

Esztergom: thermal baths (Sokollu Mustafa Pasha Baths?)

Esztergom, Katona István utca 8. (formerly Óvoda utca)

The Sokollu Mustafa Pasha Baths similarly to those preceding, are ruins trapped in a cellar, however it is a significantly larger building that extends beyond the building above.

Founder:	Sokollu Mustafa Pasha or Rüstem Pasha
Year of founding:	before 1578
Ottoman era name:	unknown
Type:	thermal baths
Groundplan type:	not possible to determine
Director of excavation:	István Horváth
Excavation year:	1952, 1968-1971, 1991
Publications:	MRT 5, pp. 123-124; Sudár 2003, p. 248

HISTORY

The few written and pictorial sources do not provide the opportunity to conclusively determine who the founder was. All we know is that Rüstem Pasha and Sokollu Mustafa Pasha also founded steam baths in the city. At the end of the 16th century, depictions of the former Óvoda Street (today Katona István Street) show in the place of today's excavated ruined baths a picture of a double bath building.

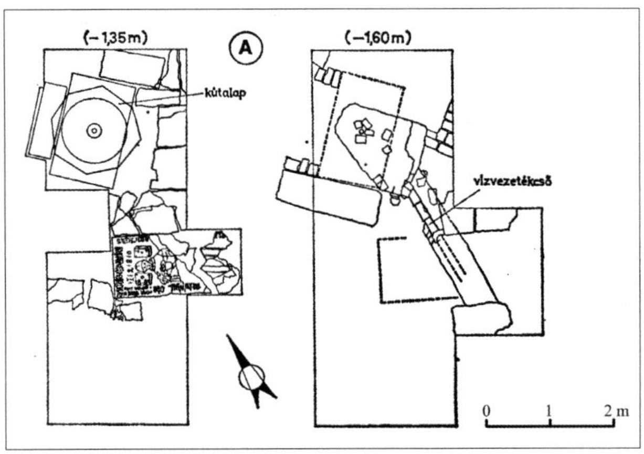

Figure 118. An excavated section of the 16th-century thermal baths in Esztergom

DESCRIPTION OF THE BUILDING

On the street, when the sewers were laid, a fountain with a water pipe beneath it was exposed. In a nearby house the ruins of the Turkish baths also came to light. In all probability, the fountain was the fountain of the spa's foyer. An octagonal area and a pool were discovered in the building (*Figure 118*).

The 1595 survey of the city suggests a northeast-southwest orientation (*Figure 119*), while the excavated ruins are rather of a southeast-northwest building (*Figure 120* 'A'). The solution to this contradiction is still awaited.

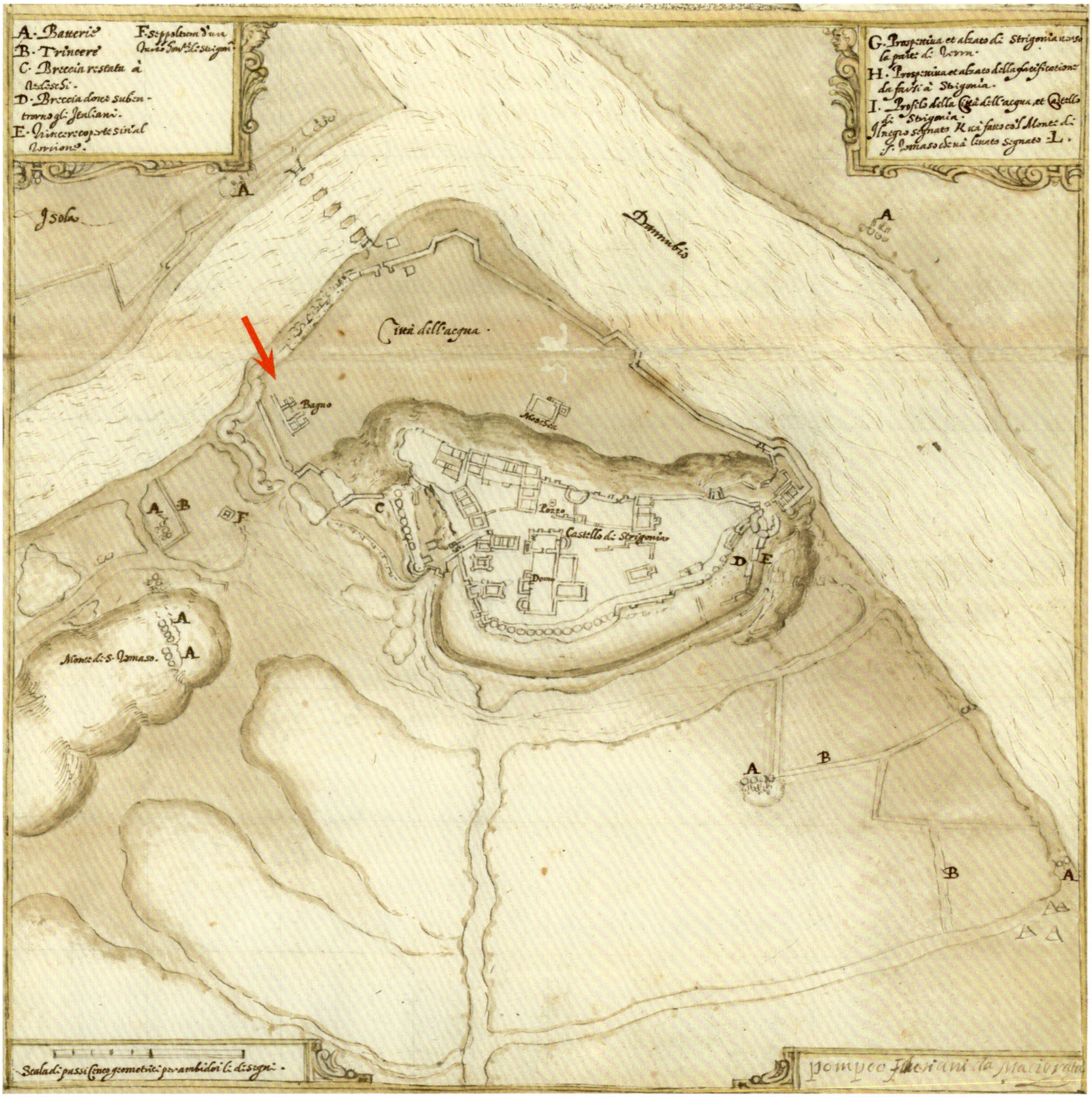

Figure 119. Section of the map created of the siege of Esztergom in 1595; the red arrow marks the baths that stood close to the Danube shore

Esztergom: thermal baths

Esztergom, József Attila tér

The small Turkish baths (later known as Mattyasovszky baths), which was completely buried in the middle of the 19th century in a fortification of the southern wall of Esztergom (the Hévízi Fortress). In recent research, the building was released from its imense covering that had preserved its four rooms and the base of the dome. The restoration and presentation of the building would enrich the city's archaeological-historical memories with a spectacular element.

Founder:	unknown
Year of founding:	after 1605
Ottoman era name:	unknown
Type:	thermal baths
Groundplan type:	single dome (H type)
Director of excavation:	István Horváth
Year of excavation:	1969 exploratory dig, 2001 partial excavation
Publications:	MRT 5, pp. 124–125; Gerelyes 2011, p. 56

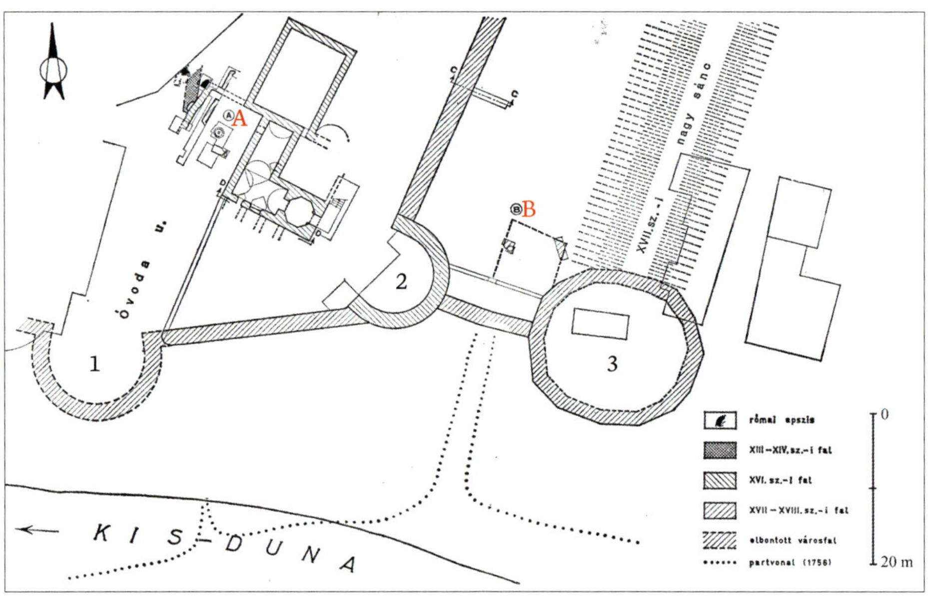

Figure 120. Esztergom, the Franciscan Bastion (1), the tower of the Hévíz baths (2), and the Hévíz fortifications (3). 'A' marks the remains of the Mustafa Pasha (?) Baths, 'B' marks the site of the small thermal baths

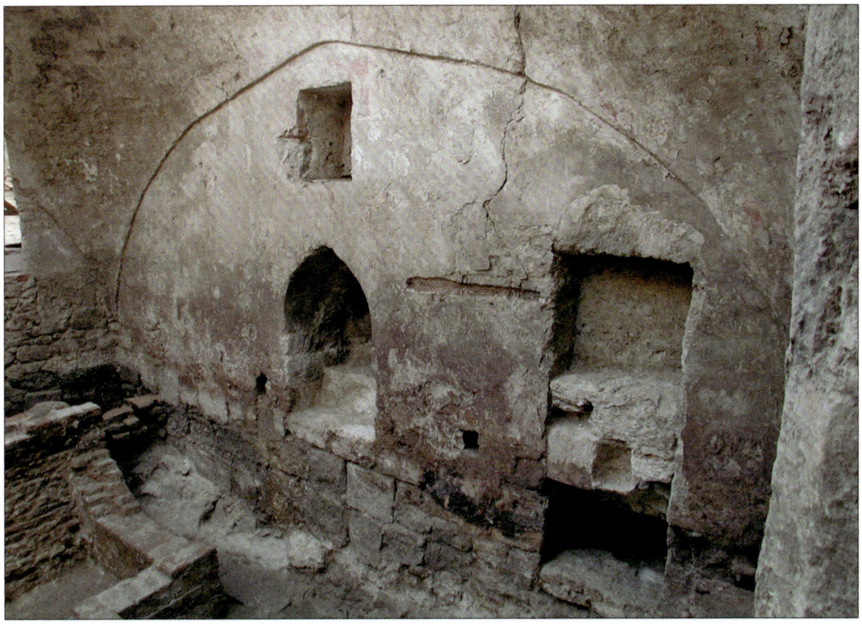

Figure 121. The line of the excavated interior walls of the Esztergom thermal baths (17th century)

DESCRIPTION OF THE BUILDING

The bath was built during the second period of Ottoman rule in the city (1605-1683), "in the moat between the Hévíz bath tower, the fortress of Hévíz, the southern wall of the city and the outer great moat, probably together with the Hévíz fortress" (see *Figure 120* 'B'). Evliya Chelebi described the poor being used. We do not know the full floor plan of the bath, and in its prime there was a small square cupola covering the room with a pool. The wall plaster in the hall is still largely visible today (*Figure 121*). A boat has been scratched into the plaster. Identification of the room is uncertain, it may be a hot room, or a private bath (*Figure 122*).

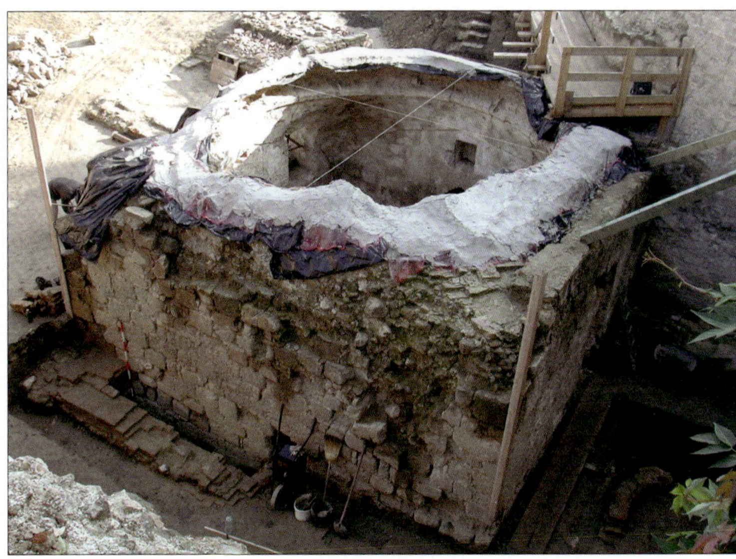

Figure 122. Exterior of the excavated 17th-century thermal baths in Esztergom

Excavated but reburied bath ruins

Double baths (Rüstem Pasha Baths?), Pest

Budapest V., Piarista köz 1.

The ruins of the spa building in the grounds of the *Sapientia* College of Theology (formerly the Piarist High School, later the Eötvös Loránd University, Faculty of Humanities) were excavated at the beginning of the 20th century, and then reburied, leaving future generations in doubt as to whether they were in fact Roman or Turkish baths. When the building was again excavated, it was found that the baths were Turkish, but they were buried once again, although they could have made an interesting sight in the refurbished Piarist courtyard (*Figure 123*).

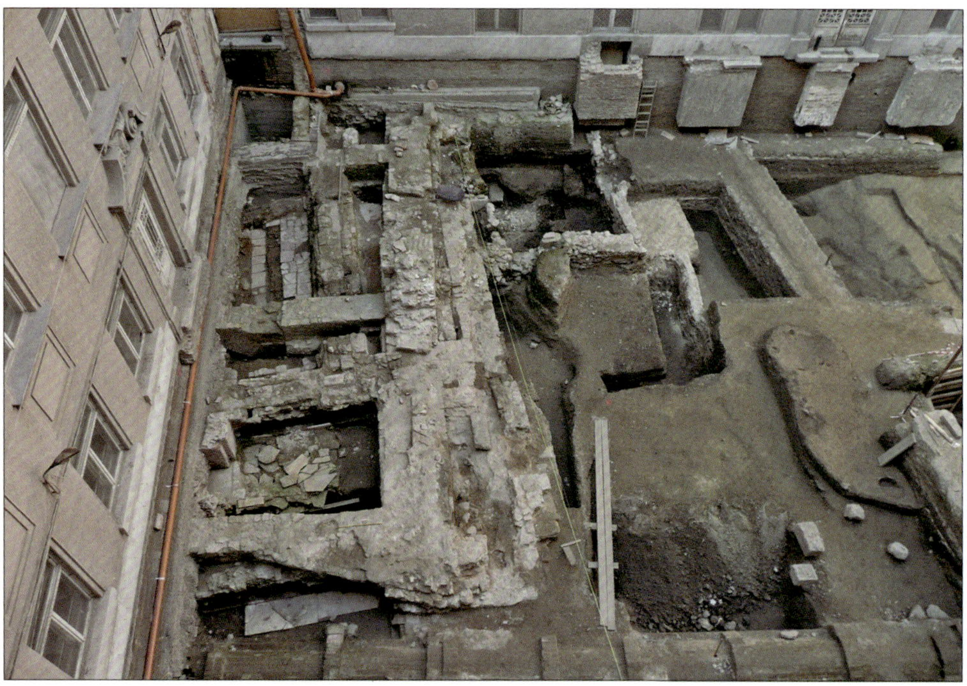

Figure 123. Pest, the double baths as they appeared during the excavation

Founder:	Rüstem Pasha?
Founded:	before 1578
Ottoman era name:	unknown
Type:	steam baths
Ground plan type:	cannot be determined (*Figure 124*)
Director of excavations:	Judit Zádor
Year of excavation:	2007
Publications:	Beszédes–Papp–Zádor 2008

Surprisingly, the ruins of the baths hidden beneath the building of the Piarist High School in Pest were never forgotten.[140] Parts of the baths were discovered at the time when the new high school was built in 1914, at which time they were identified as Turkish baths.[141] The once again buried ruins remain under the western and northern wings of the grammar school and under some of its yard. Lajos Nagy, an archaeologist at the Aquincum Museum, considered baths to be from the Roman era based on the published pictures and the nearby Roman walls. An opportunity arose to determine their age when the Piarist building was renovated in 2007 and its yard was built over. Archaeological research carried out in the courtyard and the northern wing of the building clearly showed[142] that the bath building was from the Ottoman period.

In Pest, Rüstem Pasha and Sokollu Mustafa Pasha also founded baths, as well as a public steam bath.[143] Mustafa Pasha's baths was near the pasha's mosque, which, according to Balázs Sudár, was on Ferenciek Square.[144] Consequently, the baths must be either the public baths or the Rüstem Pasha baths.

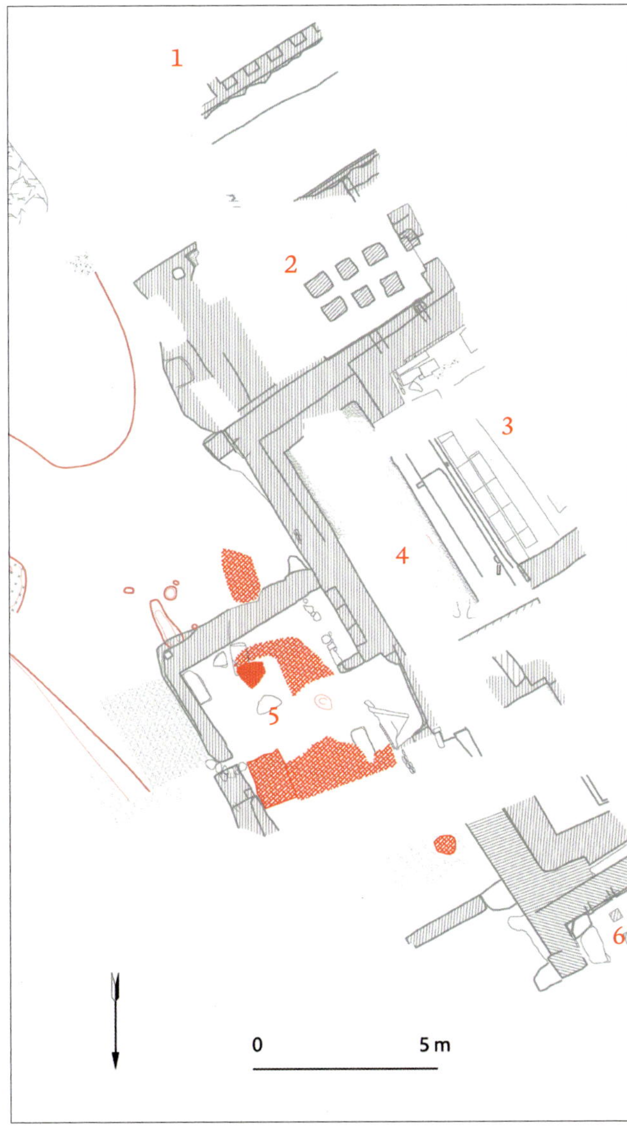

Figure 124. Pest, the floorplan of the double baths. 1. Entrance hall. 2. Warm room. 3. Hot room. 4. Cistern. 5. Heating area. 6. The remainder of the ruins of the baths

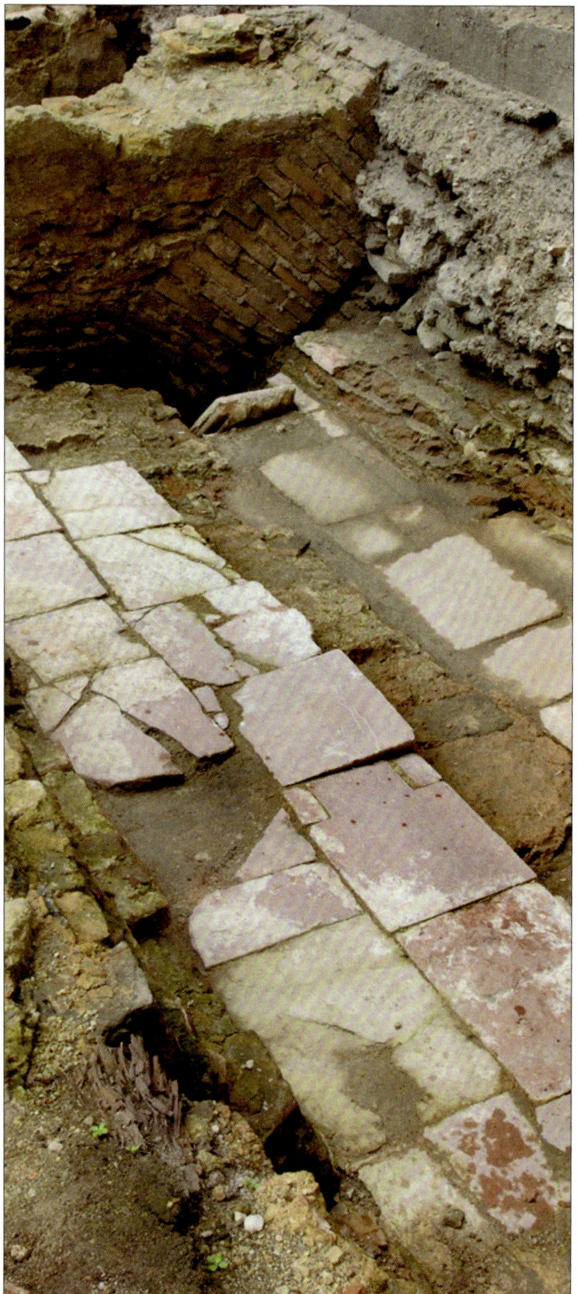

Figure 125. Pest, Ottoman era remains of marble floor in the hot area of the double baths

DESCRIPTION OF THE BUILDING

During the new excavations, the building was rediscovered in a largely destroyed state, ruined by the intrusion of large broad pillars and various modern walls. The underfloor heating system and floor of the baths were almost completely intact, and in the walls, there was a two-line plumbing system that had fed the basins of the baths.

The bath building lies northwest to southeast, and during the excavations the main parts could be identified. The entrance hall was the southernmost room of the present-day City Centre Church (a mosque in the Ottoman era). There was a glimpse of the toothed wall benches typical of the entrance hall, and a part of the floor.

The next two rooms could have belonged to the warm room, and the floor and door of the room to the north could be identified. North of this is the hot room, whose red marble floors (*Figure 125*), walls and even water pipes, have survived. The naval stone sited in the middle of the hall was covered by one of the walls of the new high school, but a small part of it was identifiable. Interestingly, the hot room's eastern end wall is further west than those of the warm rooms. Here, on the eastern edge of the building, archaeologists discovered the bottom, plastered part of a water tank. This space was cut longitudinally by a modern wall. The continuation of the water tank was traced by the diggers beneath the northern wing of the standing Piarist building, and even the boiler room to the east was found. Based on this, an interesting bath building can be reconstructed: a double bath building, but one with an uncommon arrangement, with two areas are in contact with the hot rooms.[145]

Of further interest is that alongside the stone-built walls of the baths, the parts in which the plumbing and ventilation ducts of the underfloor heating system were built are of brick. On the walls there are many places where the pink and red plaster of the Ottoman era remain.

The Toygun Pasha Baths, Buda

Budapest I., Fő utca 30.

In the inner-city area, a lot of difficulties can be encountered in exploring a building. Thus, almost completely demolished baths are hidden in the Víziváros basement of the Capuchin Church monastery buildings in Buda. After partial exploration they were reburied. Full exploration and presentation is impossible for architectural reasons.

Founder:	Toygun Pasha
Founded:	around 1555
Ottoman era name:	*Toygun Pasha Hamami* (Toygun Pasha Baths)
Type:	steam baths
Ground plan type:	single dome (H type) or star-shaped (B type) (*Figure 126*)
Director of excavations:	Győző Gerő, Katalin H. Gyürky
Year of excavation:	1972–1973
Publications:	Gerő 2003

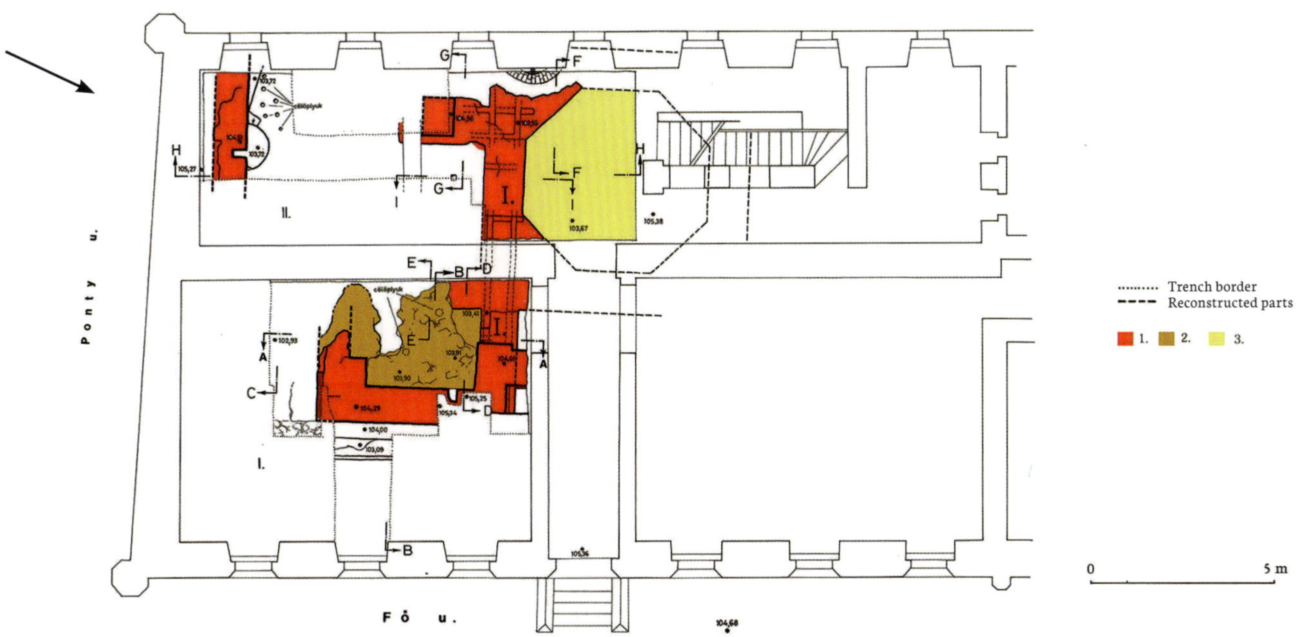

Figure 126. Buda, 1973 survey drawing of the ruins of the Toygun Pasha Baths. 1. Ottoman era walls. 2. Foundations of the floor heating. 3. Clay filling

HISTORY

The baths were built between 1553-1555 along with the mosque next to them. Since these were average Ottoman steam baths, we do not have much written information about them. Trader and diplomat Hans Dernschwam recalls the building in 1555 as being huge baths, and notes that "the most beautiful stones have been transported here from all over".[146] Among other places, marble was also transported here from the cathedral at Pécs.[147] Evliya Chelebi refers only to their existence.[148] That is confirmed by de La Vigne's[149] floor plan, but the annotated Ottoman map[150] only names the mosque. It does not appear on the Luigi Ferdinando Marsigli[151] list, but we can probably identify it as the double baths at the end of the listing. This is reinforced by de La Vigne's map, which depicts the contours of the baths in real life: in this case, square baths are shown on the map. This is interesting because the overwhelming majority of Ottoman baths in the classical era were rectangular in design. However, in the case of double baths, two rectangles were placed next to each other, so in the end we get a square floor plan just as shown on de La Vigne's map. So, it is very likely that this little-known steam bath was the only Ottoman double bath in Buda.

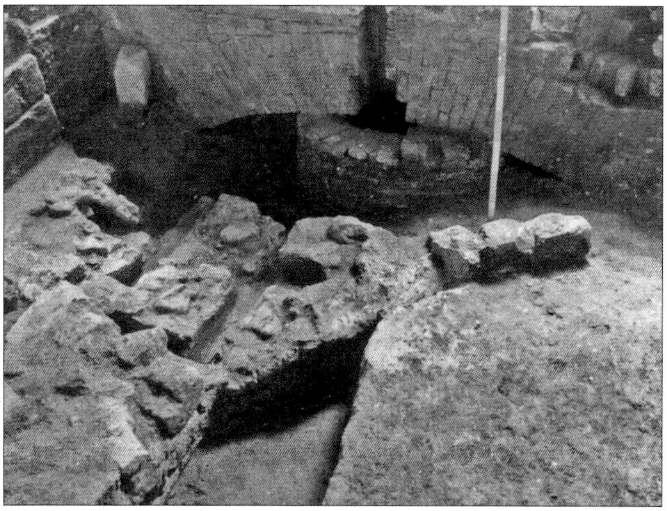

Figure 127. The Toygun Pasha Baths, probably the foundations of the hot room

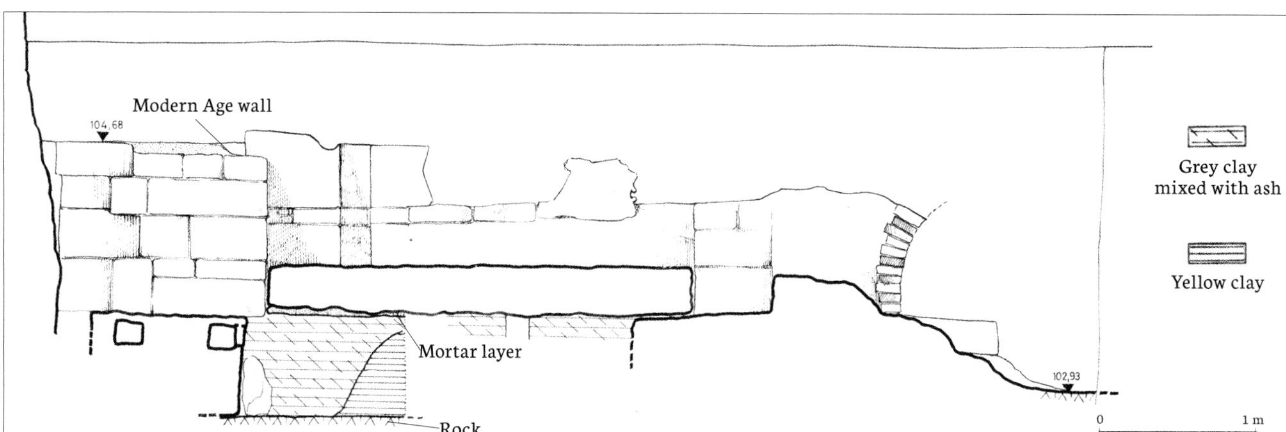

Figure 128. Survey drawing made during the excavation of the Toygun Pasha Baths

DESCRIPTION OF THE BUILDING

What do the excavation results tell us? Unfortunately, very little, but they raise a number of questions. Research in a limited area has only exposed limited, severely damaged and difficult to interpret building parts (*Figure 127–128*). The walls discovered could have once belonged to two, three or even more rooms whose shape and function is difficult to identify. The excavated ruins belonged to the foundation of the baths floor heating. Sometimes this layer was destroyed and only the stamped clay remained below it, as in the octagonal room. The unique shape of the latter indicates that it could have been the hot room. To the south of it a masonry column was found, which could be a remnant of the underfloor heating in the adjacent room.

Based on the excavations, the extent of the former baths can be determined, but there is not enough data for accurate dimensions. This section of the building on the west side of de La Vigne's map has disappeared in the Modern Age, but its northern and southernmost parts still exist (Kapucinus Street). Today's Ponty Street bordered the building, and in the east, it certainly did not reach today's Fő Street. Based on all this, the Capuchin monastery in the west certainly extended over the baths, as evidenced by the walls. The southern end wall was found alongside the southern wall of the monastery. To the east, only the eastern wall of the terrace with underfloor heating was found. Since there was no underfloor heating here, it could be that the Capuchin Building extends eastwards across the entrance hall. There is at this juncture a wall extending northwards, meaning that east of the octagonal room there were also bath rooms.

The Ferhad Pasha Baths, Pécs

Pécs, Kossuth utca 23-25.

Archaeologists often have to face the question, when they find architectural remains that will be reburied, of why they cannot be demolished if they are going to be concreted over? In archaeological-heritage conservation, it is important for the remains to be preserved even if, within the foreseeable future, there is no chance of being their being presented. These baths were researched long ago, but the surveys provide us with a lot of knowledge about the building.

Founder:	Ferhad Pasha[152]
Founder:	unknown
Ottoman era name:	*Ferhad Pasha Hamami* (Ferhad Pasha Baths)
Type:	steam baths
Ground plan type:	single dome on the male section (H type), a central dome on the female section (E type) (*Figure 129*)
Director of excavations:	Gábor Kárpáti
Year of excavation:	1984 (during the laying of gas mains, archaeological phenomena were observed)
Publications:	Szőnyi 1928; Gerő 1980, p. 111; Kárpáti 1985

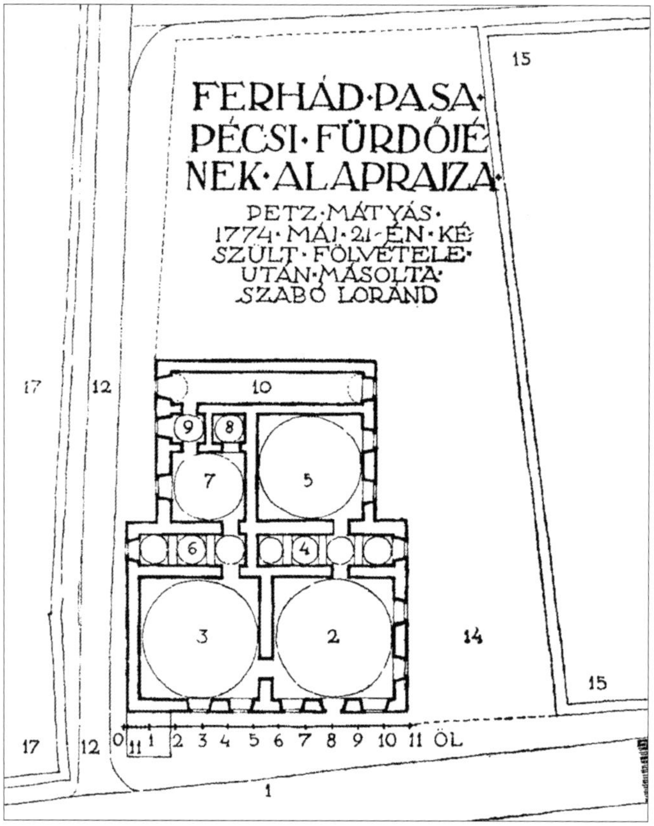

Figure 129. Pécs, survey of the Ferhad Pasha Baths from 1885

HISTORY

The floor plan of the baths is known from a survey made in 1774, and later in 1885 the ruins were surveyed when the house built above was demolished. Nearly a hundred years later, in 1984, the building was authenticated during archaeological excavations. The map by Joseph de Haüy of Pécs shows that the baths were built along the road between the Szigetvár and Buda Gate Road, and a smaller street that lay on the west side.

DESCRIPTION OF THE BUILDING

We can learn a lot about the baths from the remaining survey drawings. We can see the rooms and the roofs of the double baths. All of which describes a large double bath covered with domes. Over the western bath section there were three domes, and over the eastern there were four domes. The hot room floor layout also differs. In the western part, the double private baths (E type) solution was chosen, but the *iwans* are missing. On the east side there was a large dome covering the hot room.

The survey made in 1885 shows a more controversial picture. We find none of the regular square rooms that are indispensable for domes. However, the difference could be due to the circumstances of the survey and to the measurement technique: the 18th-century surveyor was in an easier position as he actually saw the domes, so he could base his depiction on the spectacle rather than on the specific measurements. Therefore, for the domed rooms, the 18th-century survey can be regarded as the more credible source.

The two parts of the double baths were side by side so that spaces with the same function were placed side by side. To identify the female and male parts, the orientation of the building and the ratio of the two parts to each other can serve as a reference. The western part of the building was smaller, and its entrance would have been from the small street near the baths, so this would have been the female part. The eastern part was bigger, and its entrance could only have opened from the main street, so that was the male part.

Steam baths, Babócsa

Babócsa, Basha Garden Nature Reserve (Nárciszos)

The number of the buildings shown so far has little to do with the Ottoman steam baths found in the Basha Garden (Nárciszos) in the Dráva countryside of Babócsa (*Figure 130*). The location is outside the settlement border, about one and a half kilometres east of the village, near the Rinya Water. While the buildings presented so far were built in larger Ottoman centres, these steam baths were located in one of the strongholds of Babócsa or, more precisely, in a settlement of more than four hectares with ramparts and fortresses. So far, there have been no Turkish baths in any similar settlement. From the written sources we know that there were many small fortresses with baths, but these buildings are still represented only by the Babócsa baths.

Founder:	Skender Bey of Szigetvár
Founded:	1566–1570
Ottoman era name:	unknown
Type:	steam baths
Baths floor plan type:	single dome (H type) (*Figure 131*)
Director of excavations:	Kálmán Magyar
Year of excavation:	1988
Publications:	Magyar 1990, pp. 118–128; Nagy 1990, pp. 384–389; Magyar 2002, pp. 95–97.

The warm and hot room of the baths, the toilets and the boiler house were excavated. Only the underfloor heating levels remained in the exposed rooms, neither the floor covering, nor the walls survived into the 20th century. An interesting feature of the baths is that the observed interior walls of the hot room were curved, as if the room were circular. There is no known example in Ottoman architecture, so it is more likely that they continued in a different way above floor level on the ascending walls, perhaps octagonally. Such a solution would have suited Turkish baths.

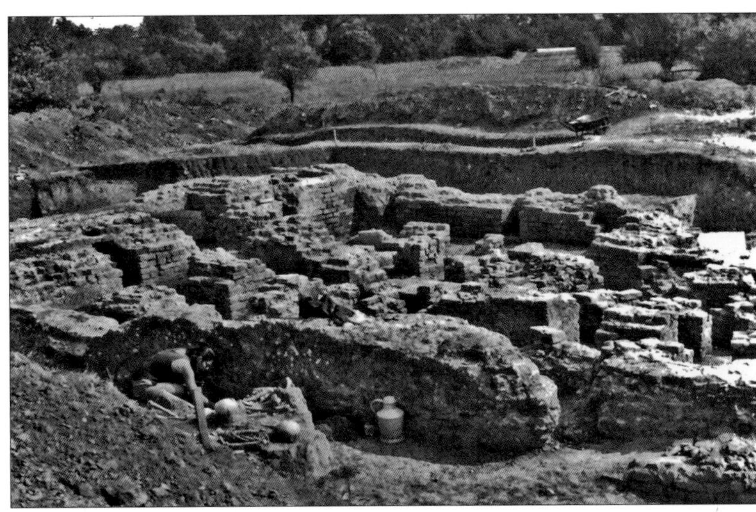

Figure 130. Babócsa, the steam baths during excavation (1988)

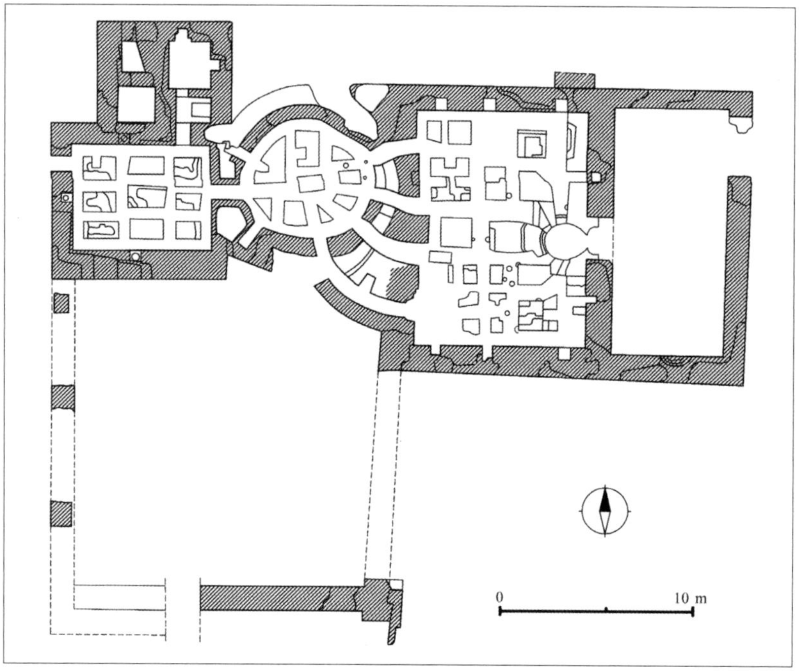

The toilets were lined up beside the warm room. The archaeologist leading the excavation from the south assumed there had been a large entrance hall, but it had to have been on the west side next to the warm room. Due to its location, it is conceivable that the explored room, whose walls were made of clay and stone, was independent of the bath. Its function cannot be determined.

During the excavations, a well that supplied the bath with water was also excavated near the building.

Figure 131. Babócsa, steam baths floorplan

Commander's Palace private baths, Babócsa

Babócsa, Basha Garden Nature Reserve (Nárciszos)

A major building was discovered during archaeological research, which was identified by the excavator as the Ottoman Palace of Command. At the eastern end of the building, baths (part of the private baths at the palace) were found, and the under the bath section, underfloor heating and the remains of the heater. Based on the partial details, an exact reconstruction of the building and the baths is not possible.

Founder:	unknown
Founded:	unknown
Ottoman era name:	unknown
Type:	steam baths
Baths floor plan type:	not possible to determine
Director of excavations:	Kálmán Magyar
Year of excavation:	1989
Publications:	Magyar 1990, pp. 128-138; Nagy 1990, pp. 389-390; Magyar 2002

Key to Abbreviations

Aqfüz	Aquincumi füzetek (Aquincum Booklets)
BFL	Budapest Főváros Levéltára (Budapest City Archive)
BL	British Library
BTM	Budapesti Történeti Múzeum (Budapest History Museum)
BTM KO	Budapesti Történeti Múzeum Középkori Osztály (Budapest History Museum, Department of the Mediaeval Era)
BudRég	Budapest Régiségei (Antiquities of Budapest)
HMI	Hadtörténeti Múzeum és Intézet (Museum and Institute of War History)
JPMÉ	Janus Pannonius Múzeum Évkönyvei (Janus Pannonius Museum Yearbooks)
KÖH	Kulturális Örökségvédelmi Hivatal (Office of Cultural Heritage Protection)
MNL	Magyar Nemzeti Levéltár (The Hungarian National Archive)
ÖStA, HHStA	Haus-, Hof- und Staatsarchiv, Wien (Austrian State Archive, Vienna)
RégFüz	Régészeti Füzetek (Archaeological Booklets)
TBM	Tanulmányok Budapest Múltjából (Studies of Budapest's Past)
TSM	Topkapı Sarayı Müzesi Arşivi (Topkapi Palace Museum Archive)

Notes

1 For more information on Evliya Chelebi, see e.g. Fodor 1990; Sudár 2012b, pp. 11-48..

2 Evliya 2002, p. 153.

3 Hegyi 2007.

4 Sudár 2012, pp. 40-49.

5 Necipoğlu 2005, p. 133.

6 Hillenbrand 2013, 21-24.

7 Kovács 2009.

8 Kováts 1966.

9 Gaál 2002.

10 Kovács-Rózsás 2010.

11 Gerelyes 1996.

12 Hatházi 1999; Hatházi-Kovács 2016.

13 Papp 2015.

14 Sudár 2012, p. 41; Sudár 2017.

15 Sudár 2014.

16 Ágoston-Sudár 2002.

17 Sudár 2013.

18 Sudár 2013, IV: Appendix: Türbék a magyar hódoltságban [*Türbes* in Ottoman Hungary], pp. 70-91.

19 *Magyar Tudomány* [Hungarian Science], September 2016, pp. 1026-1074.

20 Hancz 2016; Fodor (ed.) 2017.

21 Sinan 2014, preface by G. Necipoğlu, pp. 360-361.

22 Dernschwam 1984.

23 Evliya 2002, pp. 134-157.

24 Papp 2013.

25 Kertész 2008; Kertész-Morgós-Nagy-Szántó 2007.

26 Tóth 2010, 879-880.

27 Kuran 1980.

28 Eyice 1960, typology: pp. 108-115, figure 5.

29 Veress 1906, p.136, p.148.

30 Şahin 1994, p. 245.

31 Önge 1989, pp. 403-428.

32 Gerelyes 1979, 208, 211.

33 TSM B. 408, Fol. 18.

34 Sudár 2003.

35 BTM Engravings Archive, inv. no. 2014.9.1.

36 E.g. Evliya Chelebi (Evliya 2002, pp.147-149.)

37 Veress 1906.

38 The travel descriptions suggest that there was a bath in the palaces of the earlier pashas, but none have been found to date. (Reinhold Lubenau, in: Haraszti-Pethő 1963, p.89.).

39 Gerő 1987.

40 Published by Szőnyi 1928.

41 Sudár 2003, pp. 254-257.

42 Sudár 2003, pp. 245-247.

43 Beszédes-Papp-Zádor 2008.

44 Sudár 2003, p. 257.

45 Sudár 2003, pp. 249-250.

46 Evliya 2002 (VII. 26).

47 Gerő 1977, p. 113; Siklósi 1989; Sudár 2003, pp. 249-250.

48 Gerő 1977, pp. 112-113; Siklósi 1989, pp. 156-157.

49 On the basis of the data in Sudár 2003.

50 Kütahya 9 (Altun 1982-1982), Tire 13 (Çakmak 2002, p. 1), Belgrade 11 (Ayverdi 2000, p. 25), Skopje 12 (Ayverdi 2000, p. 346), Sarajevo 8 (Ayverdi 2000, p. 344), Prizen 2 (Ayverdi 2000, p. 343).

51 Sudár 2003.

52 Bizbirlik 2002, pp. 18-20, 33-34, 38-40, 79, 89, 175, 259, 299, 302, 304, 306, 312, 324, 327, 336, 377, 379, 407, 416, 431.

53 Gévay 1841, p. 17.

54 Sudár 2012, pp. 93-104.

55 Hegyi 1995, p. 169.

56 Hegyi 1995, p. 167.

57 TSM D7000 8b.

58 TSM D7000 9a.

59 TSM D7000 8b.

60 TSM D7000 8b.

61 Sudár 2014, p. 265.

62 Soós 1962.

63 Cf. Sudár 2014, pp. 278-279.

64 Şehitoglu 2008, p. 27.

65 E.g. Molnár 1961; Molnár 1965; Molnár 1969; Molnár 1973.

66 Hegyi 2010.

67 See in detail Papp-Lászay 2009-2010.

68 Klinghardt 1927, Abb. 12; Kanetaki 2012, figure 26.

69 Önge 1978, p. 133.

70 Önge 1978, figures 24, 25; Önge 1978, figure 27.

71 Kilich Ali Pasha Hamami in Istanbul and the Nasuh Pasha Hamami in Bursa.

72 Szőnyi 1928, p. 41.

73 Gerő 1980, figure 92.

74 In the Boyahane hamami in Erzurum the halvets are octagonal.

75 Erken 2006, plan 10.

76 Haskan 1995, p. 176.

77 The hot room of the Süleymaniye Hamami in Istanbul is 10 metres across, while that of the Rudas bath is 17 metres.

78 Önge 1989, p. 256.

79 Sinan 2014, p. 80.

80 Necipoğlu 2005, pp.158, 159.

81 Erlach 1725, Book 3, Table 1.

82 Linzbauer 1837.

83 Károlyi 1886.

84 Foerk 1918, pp. 38-48.

85 Molnár 1969; Molnár 1973.

86 Fekete 1944, pp. 94-97, 116-118.

87 Gerő 1958; Gerő 1959.

88 Molnár 1976.

89 Gerő 1980.

90 Sudár 2003.

91 In the works of Evliya Chelebi (Evliya 2002, pp. 145-146) and Edward Brown (Brown 1673, p. 96), and in the surveys and maps of Marsigli (Veress 1906, inserted after pages 136 and 138, p. 144).

92 Sudár 2003.

93 The examination was carried out by András Grynaeus. Papp-Grynaeus 2011, pp. 260-262.

94 For the surroundings of the Rudas Baths see Papp 2009.

95 The replacement of the water pipes is indicated by the completely different pipes that lay alongside: a white glazed piping connected to unglazed red material.

96 Marsigli: Veress 1906, p. 136.

97 Fehérvári 2006, figures 13-14.

98 Fehérvári 2006, pp. 26-47, 29.

99 MNL T62 No. 898.

100 For a detailed Modern Age history of the baths see Fehérvári 2006.

101 Radnainé (ed.) 2006, Fig. 13.

102 Fehérvári 2006, p. 31.

103 BFL 167/423.

104 Radnainé (ed.) 2006, figure 46.

105 Judit Lászay directed the wall excavation, the paint restoration research was carried out by Gizella Makoldy.

106 Visible, e.g. on the map by de La Vigne (BTM Engravings Archive, inv. no. 2014.9.1.), also on the map produced in 1760 (HMI GIH 67/3).

107 Brown 1673, p. 96.

108 For the adventurous history of the Császár Baths see Sudár 2003; Sudár 2006.

109 The analysis was carried out by András Grynaeus, see Papp-Grynaeus 2011, pp. 264-265.

110 Old maps of Budapest I. DVD kat. 110, BFL XV.16.d. 241, BTM 430, for dating: Rozsnyai 2008, p. 64.

111 For the Modern Age history of the baths, see Rozsnyai 2008.

112 Judit Lászay directed the wall excavation was, the paint restoration research was carried out by Gizella Makoldy.

113 It appears thus on Marsigli's map, see Veress 1906, pp. 136, 144.

114 Evliya 2002, p. 148.

115 Omichius 1582, 11a.

116 TSM D7000 9a.

117 The dendrochronological examination was carried out by András Grynaeus, see Papp-Grynaeus 2011, pp. 262-264.

118 Evliya 2002, p. 148.

119 Veress 1906, p. 136

120 Most clearly noticeable in the writings of Melchior Besolt: "Before a person goes into the bath, they find a lovely, broad room in which they can undress." (Sudár 2003, p. 228.)

121 Bor 2007.

122 Bor 2007, figure 43.

123 The floorplan of the building. Bültenmeyer's engraving (Heinrich 1873).

124 Evliya 2002, p. 148.

125 Veress 1906, p. 136.

126 Omichius, 1582, 11a.

127 Borsos 1958, p. 24.

128 TSM D7000 9A.

[129] Borsos 1958, p. 26.

[130] Gerő 1958, p. 590.

[131] Brown 1673, p. 22.

[132] Veress 1906, p. 136.

[133] Borsos 1958.

[134] Evliya 2002 (VII, pp. 66-67.)

[135] E.g. the Nasuh Pasha, Hüsnügüzel and Injirli Baths (Bursa), Kilich Ali Pasha and Arasta Baths (Istanbul), Sokollu Mehmed Pasha Baths (Lüleburgaz).

[136] Reinhold Lubenau (Haraszti-Pethő 1963, p. 89.)

[137] Veress 1906, p. 137.

[138] Evliya 2002, p. 140.

[139] Evliya 2002, p. 145.

[140] Nagy 1934, footnote 41.

[141] Friedrich 1914, p. 30.

[142] Based on the stratification and the ceramic plumbing tubes remaining in the building.

[143] Sudár 2003.

[144] Sudár 2014, pp. 446-447. At the time of the construction of the University Library, the ruins of baths buildings were said to have come to light that could be the Sokullu Mustafa's baths.

[145] For example, the Haseki Hürrem Baths in Istanbul.

[146] Dernschwam 1984, p. 498.

[147] Hegyi 2010, pp. 30, 84-85.

[148] Evliya 2002, p. 147.

[149] BTM Engravings Archive, inv. no. 1.9.2014.

[150] Veress 1906, inserted after p.138.

[151] Veress 1906, pp. 136-137.

[152] The founder, Ferhad Pasha, is difficult to identify with the person known from Ottoman Hungary. For this problem, see: Gere-Sudár 2011.

Bibliography

Ágoston-Sudár 2002

Ágoston G. - Sudár B.: *Gül Baba és a magyarországi bektasi dervisek.* [Gül Baba and the Hungarian Bektashi Dervishes] Budapest: Terebess Kiadó, 2002.

Altun 1981-1982

A. Altun: Kütahya'nın türk devrimimarisi. In: *Kütahya.* Istanbul, Kütahya Belediyesi: İstanbul Üniversitesi Edebiyat Fakültesi, Sanat Tarihi Enstitüsü, 1981-1982, pp. 171-700.

Ayverdi 2000

E. H. Ayverdi: *Avrupa'da Osmanlı Mimârî Eserleri. Yugoslavya.* III. kitap. Istanbul: İstanbul Fetih Cemiyeti, Bilmen Basımevi, 2000.

Beszédes-Papp-Zádor 2008

Beszédes J. - Papp A. - Zádor J.: Római kori védmű és török fürdő a pesti belvárosban. [Roman Era Defences and Turkish Baths in the City of Pest] *AqFüz* 14 (2008), pp. 165-202.

Bizbirlik 2002

A. Bizbirlik: *16. yüzyıl ortalarında Diyarbekir beylerbeyliğinde vakıflar: 972 tahriri ışığında.* Ankara: Türk Tarih Kurumu, 2002.

Bor 2007

Bor F.: *A Rác fürdő művészettörténeti dokumentációja.* [Documentation of the Art History of the Rác Baths] Unpublished manuscript, 2007.

Borsos 1958

Borsos B.: A Király fürdő helyreállítása. [The Restoration of the Király Baths] *Műemlékvédelem* 2 (1958), 23-34.

Brown 1673

E. Brown: *A Brief Account of Some Travels in Hungaria.* London: T. R. for Benj. Tooke, 1673.

Çakmak 2002

C. Çakmak: *Tirehamamları.* Ankara: Türk Tarih Kurumu, 2002.

Dernschwam 1984

H. Dernschwam: *Erdély. Besztercebánya. Törökországi útinapló.* [Travel Journal from Transylvania, Besztercebánya. Turkey] (ed.) Tardy L. Bibliotheca Historica. Budapest: Európa Könyvkiadó, 1984.

Erken 2006

S. Erken: Edirne hamamları. *Vakıflar Dergisi* 10 (2006), pp. 403-419.

ERLACH 1725

J. B. Fischer von Erlach: *Entwurff einer historischen Architectur.* Leipzig, 1725.

EVLIYA 2002

Evliyâ Çelebi b. Derviş Mehemmed Zillî: *Evliyâ Çelebi Seyahatnâmesi.* Topkapı Sarayı Kütüphanesi Revan 1457 Numaralı Yazmanın Transkripsiyonu - Dizini. 6. Kitap. Haz. Seyyid Ali Kahraman-Yücel Dağlı. Istanbul: Yapı Kredi Yayınları, 2002.

EYICE 1960

S. Eyice: Iznik'de "Büyük Hamam" ve Osmanlı devri hamamları hakkında bir deneme. In: *Tarih Dergisi* 11/15, 1960, pp. 99-120.

FEHÉRVÁRI 2006

Fehérvári Z.: A fürdő kiépítése a török kiűzésétől a 19. század végéig. In: RADNAINÉ (ed.) 2006, pp. 26-47.

FEKETE 1944

Fekete L.: *Budapest a török korban.* [Budapest in the Ottoman Era] Budapest: Királyi Magyar Egyetemi Nyomda, 1944.

FODOR (ed.) 2017

Fodor P. (ed.): Szulejmán szultán Szigetváron. A szigetvári kutatások 2013-2016 között. [Sultan Süleyman in Szigetvár. Research between 2013-2016] Pécs: Pannon Castrum Kft., 2017.

FODOR 1990

Fodor P.: Evlia Cselebi útleírása. [Travelogue of Evliya Chelebi] *Keletkutatás* Autumn 1990, 37-55.

FOERK 1918

Foerk E.: *Török emlékek Magyarországon.* [Ottoman Remains in Hungary] (A Budapesti Magyar Állami Felső Építő Ipariskola 1917-ik évi szünidei felvételei VI.) [Holiday period records of the Budapest Hungarian State Building Industry High School for 1917, VI] Budapest: Korvin Testv. Grafikai Intézet, 1918.

FRIEDRICH 1914

Friedrich E.: A *budapesti piarista telek története.* [The History of the Budapest Piarist Site.] Budapest: Stephaneum Nyomda, 1914.

GAÁL 2002

Gaál A.: Török palánkvárak a buda-eszéki út Tolna megyei szakaszán. [Ottoman Palisade Forts on the Tolna County Section of the Buda-Eszék Route] In: Gerelyes I. - Kovács Gy. (eds) *A hódoltság régészeti kutatása.* [Archaeological Research of Ottoman Hungary] Budapest: Magyar Nemzeti Múzeum, 2002, pp. 99-102.

GERE-SUDÁR 2011

Gere L. - Sudár B.: A pécsi Ferhád dzsámi. [The Ferhad Mosque in Pécs] *ArchÉrt* 136 (2011), pp. 269-296.

GERELYES 1979

Gerelyes I.: Török hagyatéki összeírások, mint kultúrtörténeti források. [Legacy of the Ottoman Censuses as Cultural History Sources] *TBM* 21 [Studies from the Past of Budapest 21] (1979), pp. 200-218.

Gerelyes 1996

Gerelyes I.: Török építkezések Gyulán (1566-1695). In: Szatmári I.- Gerelyes I. (eds) *Tanulmányok a gyulai vár és uradalma történetéhez.* [Studies on the History of Gyula Castle and its Estates] Gyulai füzetek 8 [Booklets from Gyula 8]. Gyula: Békés Megyei Levéltár, 1996, pp. 101-124.

Gerelyes 2011

Gerelyes I.: Ottoman Architecture in Hungary: new discoveries and perspectives for research. In: M. Hartmuth (ed.) *Proceedings of the international conference "Centers and peripheries in Ottoman architecture: rediscovering a Balkan heritage".* Sarajevo: Cultural Heritage without Border. Regional office Sarajevo, 2011, pp. 50-59.

Gerő 1958

Gerő Gy.: A törökkori Király fürdő. A Kakas kapu fürdője I. [The King's Baths in the Ottoman Era. The Cockerel Gate Baths] *BudRég* 18 (1958), pp. 587-599.

Gerő 1959

Gerő Gy.: Király fürdő. [The King's Baths] *RégFüz* 11 (1959), pp. 57-58.

Gerő 1963

Gerő Gy.: A török kori Király fürdő. 2. közlemény [The King's Baths in the Ottoman Era 2. Statement]. *BudRég* 20 (1963), pp. 137-154.

Gerő 1968

Gerő Gy.: A budai pasák vári palotája. [The Castle Palace of the Buda Pashas] *Budapest* 6/9 (1968), p. 42.

Gerő 1972

Gerő Gy.: Valide szultána fürdő. [The Valide Sultan Baths] In: Dercsényi D. - Voit P. (eds) *Heves megye műemlékei II. Eger Város műemlékei.* [Historic Monuments of Heves County II. Ancient Monuments of Eger Town] Budapest: Akadémiai Kiadó, 1972, pp. 276-280.

Gerő 1977

Gerő Gy.: Istolni Belgrád építészeti emlékei. [Architectural Relics of Royal White Castle] In: Kralovánszky A. (ed.) *Székesfehérvár évszázadai* III. [Székesfehérvár Centuries III] Székesfehérvár: István Király Múzeum 1977, pp. 112-117.

Gerő 1980

Gerő Gy.: *Az oszmán-török építészet Magyarországon.* [Ottoman Architecture in Hungary] Budapest: Akadémiai Kiadó, 1980.

Gerő 1987

Gerő, Gy.: Das neuerdings Freigelegte Memi paşa-Bad in Pécs. In: *Ars Turcica. Akten des VI. Internationalen Kongresses für Türkische Kunst München vom 3. bis 7. September 1979.* München: Maris, 1987, pp. 219-225.

Gerő 1999

Gerő, Gy.: The Residence of the Pasha's in Hungary and the Recently Discovered Pashasaray from Buda. In: Déroche, F. (ed.) *Art Turc - Türkisch Art. 10th International Congress of Türkisch Art - 10 Congrès international d'art turc. Actes-Proceedings.* Geneve, 1995. Genève: Fondation Max Van Berchem, 1999, pp. 353-360.

Gerő 2003

Gerő Gy.: A buda-vízivárosi Tojgun pasa dzsámi és a Tojgun pasa Mahalle. [The Toygun Pasha Mosque and the Toygun Pasha Mahalle in Buda-Víziváros] *BudRég* 37 (2003), pp. 197–208.

Gévay 1841

Gévay A.: *A budai pasák.* [The Buda Pashas] Vienna, 1841.

Hancz 2016

Hancz E.: *Az oszmán kori Szigetvár.* [Szigetvár of the Ottoman Era] Szigetvár: Szülőföld Könyvkiadó, 2016.

Haraszti–Pethő 1963

Haraszti S. – Pethő T.: *Útikalandok a régi Magyarországon* [Adventurous Journeys in Old Hungary]. Budapest: Táncsics Kiadó, 1963.

Haskan 1995

M. N. Haskan: *Istanbul hamamları.* Istanbul: Türkiye Turing ve Otomobil Kurumu Yayınları, 1995.

Hatházi 1999

Hatházi G.: Csókakő, a török végvár. [Csókakő, the Last Ottoman Castle] In: Béni K. (ed.) *A 700 éves Csókakő.* [700 Years of Csókakő] Csókakő: Csókakő község Önkormányzata, 1999, pp. 72–73.

Hatházi–Kovács 2016

Hatházi G. – Kovács Gy.: Újabb kutatások a csókakői várban. [Recent Research in Csókakő Castle] *Castrum* 2016, pp. 111–130.

Hegyi 1995

Hegyi K.: *Török berendezkedés Magyarországon* [Ottoman Settlements in Hungary]. Budapest: História-MTA Történettudományi Intézete, 1995.

Hegyi 2007

Hegyi K.: *A török hódoltság várai és várkatonasága* I–III. [The Castles and Castle Troops of the Ottoman Occupation I-III] Budapest: História-MTA Történettudományi Intézete, 2007.

Hegyi 2010

Hegyi K.: *Török források Pécs 16. századi történetéhez.* [Ottoman Sources in the 16th century History of Pécs] Pécs: Pécs Története Alapítvány, 2010.

Heinrich 1873

J. N. Heinrich: *Das Raitzenbad zu Ofen.* Leipzig: Weber, 1873.

Hillenbrand 2013

R. Hillenbrand: *Islamic Architecture.* Edinburgh: Edinburgh University Press, 2013.

Hunfalvy 1859

Hunfalvy J.: *Pesth und Ofennebst Umgegend. Dargestellt in malerischen Originalansichten, nach der Natur aufgenommen von Ludwig Rohbock, in Stahl gestochen von den ausgezeichnetsten Künstlern unserer Zeit.* Mit historisch-topographischem Text. [Mit 24 Stahlstichen.] (n. 8-r. 306 l.) Pest: Lauffer u. Stolp, 1859.

KANETAKI 2012

E. Kanetaki: Yunanistan'daki Osmanlı Hamamları: Tarihleri ve Mimarileri Hakkında Çalışmalara Bir Katkı. In: Ergin, N. (der.) *Anadolu Medeniyetlerinde Hamam Kültürü: Mimari, Tarih ve Imgelem.* Istanbul: Koç Üniversitesi Yayınları, 2012, pp. 269-316.

KÁROLYI 1886

Károlyi Á.: *Buda és Pest visszavívása 1686-ban.* [Recapturing Buda and Pest in 1686] Budapest: Hornyánszky, 1886.

KÁRPÁTI 1985

Kárpáti G.: Pécs-Kossuth u. 23-25. *RégFüz* 38 (1985), p. 112.

KERTÉSZ 2008

Kertész R.: Másodjára száraz lábbal. Szolnok hódoltság kori folyami átkelőinek régészeti kutatása. [Second Time with Dry Feet. Archaeological Research of the Ottoman Age River Crossings of Szolnok's Settlements.] In: Ilon G. (ed.): *Régészeti nyomozások Magyarországon.* [Archaeological Enquiries in Hungary] Budapest: Martin Opitz Kiadó, 2008, pp. 255-274.

KERTÉSZ -MORGÓS-NAGY-SZÁNTÓ 2007

Kertész R. - Morgós A. - Nagy D. - Szántó Zs.: In: Gömöri J. (ed.) *Az erdő és a fa régészete és néprajza.* [The Forest and Wood Archaeology and Ethnography] Sopron: MTA VEAB Soproni Tudós Társasága, 2007, pp. 145-178.

KLINGHARDT 1927

K. Klinghardt: *Die TürkischeBäder.* Stuttgart: Julius Hoffmann, 1927.

KOVÁCS 2009

Gy. Kovács: Ottoman Military Architecture in Hungary. In: Dávid, G.- Gerelyes, I. (eds) *Thirteenth International Congress of Turkish Art. Budapest 2007.* Budapest: Hungarian National Museum, 2009, pp. 375-392.

KOVÁCS-RÓZSÁS 2010

Kovács Gy. - Rózsás M.: A barcsi török vár és környéke. Újabb kutatások [The Ottoman Castle in Barcs and its Surroundings. New Research] (1999-2009). In: Benkő E. - Kovács Gy. (eds) *A középkor és a kora újkor régészete Magyarországon / Archaeology of the Middle Ages and Early Modern Period in Hungary* I-II. Budapest: Magyar Tudományos Akadémia Régészeti Intézete, 2010, II. pp. 621-642.

KOVÁTS 1966

Kováts V.: Sziget várának kutatástörténetéhez. [For the Research History of Sziget Castle] In: *JPMÉ* 1966, pp. 207-255.

KURAN 1980

A. Kuran: Anatolian-SeljukArchitecture. In: Akurgal, E. (ed.) *The Art and Architecture of Turkey.* New York: Rizzoli International Publications 1980, pp. 80-110.

LÁSZAY-PAPP 2005

Lászay J. - Papp A.: Régészeti feltárás és falkutatás a Rudas fürdőben. [Archaeological Exploration and Wall Research at the Rudas Baths] In: Kisfaludi J. (ed.) *Régészeti kutatások Magyarországon 2004.* [Archaeological Research in Hungary 2004] Budapest: Kulturális Örökségvédelmi Hivatal - Magyar Nemzeti Múzeum, 2005, pp. 73-90.

Lászay-Papp 2006

Lászay J. - Papp A.: A régészeti és épületkutatások eredményei a Rudas fürdőben [Archaeological and Architectural Research Results in the Rudas Baths], 2004-2005. In: Radnainé (ed.) 2006, pp. 61-83.

Lászay-Papp 2008

Lászay J. - Papp A.: Kutatások a budafelhévízi fürdőkben. [Research in the Baths of Budafelhéviz] In: Kisfaludi Júlia (ed.) *Régészeti kutatások Magyarországon 2007* [Archaeological Research in Hungary 2007]. Budapest: Kulturális Örökségvédelmi Hivatal - Magyar Nemzeti Múzeum 2008, pp. 63-84.

Lászay-Papp 2009

G. Lászay J. - Papp A.: A budai török fürdők kutatása az évezred elején. [Researching Turkish Baths in Buda at the Beginning of the Millennium] *Műemlékvédelem* 53/5 (2009), pp. 290-316.

Linzbauer 1837

F. X. Linzbauer: *Die warmen Heilquellen der Haupstadt Ofen im Königreiche Ungarn.* Pest: Hartleben, 1837.

Magyar 1990

Magyar K.: Babócsa története a honfoglalástól a mohácsi vészig.[Babócsa's history from the Hungarian Conquest to the Bane of Mohács.] In: Magyar K. (ed.) *Babócsa története. Tanulmányok a község történetéből.* [The History of Babócsa: Studies of the Community's History] Babócsa: Polgármesteri Hivatal, 1990.

Magyar 2002

Magyar K.: Babócsa-Nárciszos. Török hódoltság kori települések régészeti emlékei. [Archaeological Remains of settlements in the Ottoman Occupation.] In: Gerelyes I.- Kovács Gy. (eds) *A hódoltság régészeti kutatása.* [Archaeological Research into the Occupation] Budapest: Magyar Nemzeti Múzeum, 2002, pp. 91-98.

Maráz-Papp 2005

Maráz B. - Papp A.: Régészeti kutatások a Rác fürdő és a tabáni késő La Tène kori fazekastelep területén. [Archaeological Investigations on the Territories of Rác Bath and the Late La Tène Period Pottery Workshop of Tabán] In: Kisfaludi J. (ed.) *Régészeti kutatások Magyarországon 2005.* [Archaeological Research in Hungary 2005]. Budapest: Kulturális Örökségvédelmi Hivatal - Magyar Nemzeti Múzeum 2006, pp. 109-124.

Molnár 1961

Molnár J.: A budai Velibej fürdő építéstörténete. [The Architectural History of the Veli Bey Baths of Buda] *Építés- és Közlekedéstudományi Közlemények* 1961/4, pp. 605-621.

Molnár 1965

Molnár J.: A Valide Szultana fürdőromtípus eredete. [The Origins of the Valide Sultan Baths Ruin Type] *Műemlékvédelem* 9/1 (1965), pp. 39-41.

Molnár 1969

Molnár J.: A Rudas gyógyfürdő építéstörténete. [The Architectural History of the Rudas Baths] *Műemlékvédelem* 13/1 (1969), pp. 22-28.

Molnár 1973

Molnár J.: A budai Rác-gyógyfürdő. [The Rác Spa Baths in Buda] *Műemlékvédelem* 17/1 (1973), pp. 27-29.

Molnár 1976

Molnár J.: *A török világ emlékei Magyarországon.* [Relics of the Ottoman World in Hungary] Budapest: Corvina, 1976.

MRT 5

Horváth I. - Kelemen M. - Torma I.: *Esztergom és a Dorogi járás. Komárom megye régészeti topográfiája.* [Archaeological topography of Komárom county. Esztergom and the Dorog district] Magyarország Régészeti Topográfiája 5. [The Archaeological Topography of Hungary 5] Budapest: Akadémiai Kiadó, 1979.

Nagy 1934

Nagy L.: Pest város eredete: előzetes jelentés az eskütéri ásatásokról. [Origins of the City of Pest: preliminary report on the Eskütér excavations] *TBM* 3 [Studies of Budapest's Past 3] (1934), pp. 7-24.

Nagy 1990

Nagy G.: A Basakert építészeti öröksége, romhelyreállítás a Nárciszosban. [The Architectural Legacy of Basha Gardens and the Restoration of the Ruins in Nárciszos] In: Magyar K. (ed.) *Babócsa története. Tanulmányok a község történetéből.* [History of Babócsa. Studies of the Community's History] Babócsa: Polgármesteri Hivatal, 1990.

Necipoğlu 2005

G. Necipoğlu: *The Age of Sinan. Architectural Culture in the Ottoman Empire.* London: Reaktion, 2005.

Omichius 1582

Francisci Omichii Beschreibung Einer Legation und Reise, von Wien aus Ostereich auff Constantinopel: durch den Wolgebornen Herrn ... David Ungnadn ... auß Röm. Kaiserl. Maist. Befehl an den türkischen Kaiser anno 72 verricht. Güstrow: Ferber, 1582.

Önge 1978

Y. Önge: Eski Türk hamamlarında aydınlatma. *Vakıflar Dergisi* 12 (1978), pp. 121-135.

Önge 1989

Y. Önge: Sinan'ın inşa ettiği hamamlar. *Vakıf Haftası* 6 (1989), pp. 255-272.

Papp 2009

Papp A.: A törökkori Tabán kialakulása - az újabb régészeti adatok tükrében. [The Formation of the Ottoman Taban - In the Light of Recent Archaeological Data] *Urbs. Magyar Várostörténeti Évkönyv* 4 (2009), pp. 95-114.

Papp 2013

Papp A.: Rövid összefoglaló a budai pasák palotájáról. [A Brief Summary of the Palace of the Pashas of Buda] *BudRég* 46 (2013), pp. 167-185.

Papp 2015

Papp A.: Török kori lőpormalom Budán. [The Gunpowder Mill in Ottoman Era Buda] In: *Keletkutatás* Spring 2015, pp. 105-113.

Papp-Grynaeus 2011

Papp A. - Grynaeus A.: Budapest török fürdőinek kormeghatározása. [Determining the Age of the Turkish Baths of Budapest] *BudRég* 44 (2011), pp. 259-273.

Papp–Lászay 2009-2010

Papp A. - Lászay J.: A budai török fürdők építészete az újabb kutatások tükrében. [The Building of the Turkish Baths of Buda in the Light of Recent Research] I: Építéstechnika - építészeti elemek. [I: Construction technology - architectural elements.] *BudRég* pp. 42-43 (2009-2010), pp. 121-149.

Radnainé (ed.) 2006

Radnainé Keresztes M. (ed.): *Rudas. Gyógyfürdő - Termal Bath - Heilbad.* [Rudas Spa - Thermal Bath] Budapest: Budapest Gyógyfürdői és Hévizei Rt. kiadó, 2006.

Rózsa 1963

Rózsa Gy.: *Budapest régi látképei (1493-1800).* [Old Sights of Budapest 1493-1800] Budapest: Akadémiai Kiadó, 1963.

Rozsnyai 2008

Rozsnyai J.: A Császár fürdő építésének története a 19-20. században. [The Architectural History of the Császár Baths in the 19th-20th Centuries.] In: Marótzky K. (ed.) *Hild József építészete. Tanulmányok az építész halálának 140. évfordulójára.* [The Architecture of József Hild, Studies on the 140th Anniversary of the Architect's Death] Budapest: Terc, 2008, pp. 63-76.

Şahin 1994

K. Şahin: Deniz hamamları. In: *Vakıflar Dergisi* 23 (1994), pp. 243-254.

Şehitoğlu 2008

E. Şehitoğlu: *The Historic Hammams of Bursa.* Istanbul: Tarih Vakfı Yurt Yayınları, 2008.

Siklósi 1988

Siklósi Gy.: Székesfehérvár, Güzeldzse Rüsztem pasa fürdő. [Székesfehérvár, the Güzelje Rüstem Pasha Baths] *RégFüz* 41 (1988), p. 104.

Siklósi 1989a

Siklósi Gy.: A székesfehérvári Güzeldzse Rüsztem pasa fürdő. [The Güzelje Rüstem Pasha Baths of Székesfehérvár] *Műemlékvédelem* 33/3 (1989), pp. 154-159.

Siklósi 1989b

Siklósi Gy.: Székesfehérvár, Güzeldzse Rüsztem pasa fürdő. [Székesfehérvár, the Güzelje Rüstem Pasha Baths] *RégFüz* 42 (1989), p.90.

Siklósi 1990

Siklósi Gy.: Székesfehérvár, Güzeldzse Rüsztem pasa fürdő. [Székesfehérvár, the Güzelje Rüstem Pasha Baths] *RégFüz* 43 (1990), p.72.

Siklósi 2013

Siklósi Gy.: *A törökkori Székesfehérvár.* [Székesfehérvár in the Ottoman Era] Székesfehérvár: MH Összhaderőnemi Parancsnokság Tudományos Tanács, 2013.

Sinan 2014

Sinan's autobiographies. Five Sixteenth-century Texts. Ed. with preface by G. Necipoğlu. Leiden-Boston: Brill, 2014.

Soós 1962

Soós I.: Újabb adatok az egri török fürdőről és iskoláról. [Recent Data on the Turkish Bath and School in Eger] *Az egri vár híradója* 4 [Eger Castle News 4] (1962), pp. 23-27.

Sudár 2003

Sudár B.: Török fürdők a hódoltságban. [Turkish Baths in Ottoman Hungary] *Történelmi Szemle* 44/3-4 (2003), pp. 213-263.

Sudár 2006

Sudár B.: Mikor épült a Császár fürdő? Egy török kronogramma nyomában.[When were the Császár Baths built? Following an Ottoman Chronogram] *Keletkutatás* Spring 2002-Autumn 2006, pp. 189-200.

Sudár 2012

Sudár B.: Az oszmánok és Magyarország mentális meghódítása. [The Ottomans and the Mental Conquest of Hungary.] In: Ács P. - Székely J. (eds) *Identitás és kultúra a török hódoltság korában* [Identity and Culture in the Era of Ottoman Occupation]. Budapest: Balassi Kiadó, 2012, pp. 40-49.

Sudár 2013

Sudár B.: *A pécsi Idrisz baba-türbe.* [The Mausoleum of Idris Baba in Pécs] Budapest: Forster Gyula Nemzeti Örökséggazdálkodási és Szolgáltatási Központ, 2013.

Sudár 2014

Sudár B.: *Dzsámik és mecsetek a hódolt Magyarországon.* [Mosques and Minarets in Ottoman Hungary] Budapest: MTA Bölcsészettudományi Kutatóközpont Történettudományi Intézet, 2014.

Sudár 2017

Sudár B.: Dzsámivá alakított templomok a hódoltságban. [Churches Transformed into Mosques in Ottoman Hungary] In: Ittzés G. (ed.) *Viszály és együttélés. Vallások és felekezetek a török hódoltság korában.* [Conflict and Coexistence, Religious Belief and the Church in the Ottoman Occupation Era] Budapest: Universitas Kiadó, 2017, pp. 381-406.

Szőnyi 1928

Szőnyi O.: Ferhád pasa fürdője Pécsett. [The Pasha Ferhad Baths in Pécs] *História* 1/2 (1928), p.37.

Tóth 2010

Tóth J. A.: Adatok a kora újkori közép-Duna-medencei hajók régészetéhez. [Data for the Archeology of Early Modern Central Danube Basin Ships] In: Benkő E. - Kovács Gy. (eds) *A középkor és a kora újkor régészete Magyarországon / Archaeology of the Middle Ages and the Early Modern Period in Hungary* I-II. Budapest: Magyar Tudományos Akadémia Régészeti Intézete, 2010, II. pp. 871-883.

Veress 1906

Veress E.: Gróf Marsigli Alajos Ferdinánd olasz hadi mérnök jelentései és térképei Budavár 1684-1686-iki ostromairól, visszafoglalásáról és helyrajzáról. [Count Ferdinand Alajos Marsigli's Italian Army Engineer Reports and Maps of the Sieges, Recapture and Topography of the Buda Castle, 1684-1686] *BudRég* 9 (1906), pp. 103-170.

GLOSSARY

barrel vault - Semi-circular vault.

bey - Ottoman honorary title for a regional governor in the 16th and 17th centuries.

Blue Mosque - The Sultan Ahmed mosque in Istanbul, built between 1609-17. By Sultan Ahmed I, close to the Aya sofya.

Byzantine Empire - The eastern half of the Roman Empire. Constantinople (later Istanbul) was its capital; it fell under Ottoman Empire control in 1453.

caravanserai - See *han.*

de La Vigne, Marcel - A military engineer associated with the preparation of surveys of several Hungarian castles (1684-86), including a map and visual representation of the area around Buda and Pest.

Dernschwam, Hans - A merchant from the Czech kingdom (1494-1568/69) who acted as ambassador for King Ferdinand I to Sultan Suleiman several times. He kept a journal during his travels.

devshirme - Child tax, through which Christian children came to the Sultan's court for training and education. These people later became military and civilian officials.

dizdar - Commander of a fortress or castle.

Evliya Chelebi - Ottoman world traveller (1611-84), amongst other places, he travelled in the occupied territories. He documented some of his travels, providing one of the best sources for the period.

friday mosque - Higher ranking islamic place of worship, where Friday prayers are usually held.

göbek tashi - 'Naval stone', a raised part at the centre of the hot room of Turkish steam baths on which people could lay or sit.

grand vizier - The highest rank, just below the Sultan in the Ottoman Empire.

Hagia Sophia - A church built by the emperor Justinian between 532-537 that can still be seen today in Istanbul. Following the taking of Constantinople it was converted into a mosque, today it is a museum. On the wall there is a depiction of the Hungarian wife of the emperor, Piroska 1 (Daughter of King Laszlo I, a princess).

halvet - A smaller, private bath in a small area of the baths in which just a few people can bathe at any one time.

hamam - Steam baths.

han - Caravanserai: a place frequented by travellers and traders that was used both as a venue for trade and as accommodation.

Haüy, Joseph de - The emperor's military engineer, during the war of re-conquest he completed surveys of several castles, e.g. Buda, Pécs.

hypocaustum - An underfloor heating system.

ilija - Thermal baths.

iwan - Open on one side, closed on three other sides, a covered building part often used as an architectural solution for gates.

Iznik - The city of Anatolya where high quality feance ceramics and objects of art were manufactured in the 15th-16th centuries.

janissary - An Ottoman mercenary foot soldier.

kaplija - Thermal bath.

külliye - A building complex in which the various elements are designed and built together.

madrasa - Institution of higher education.

mahalle - An area in a settlement.

maktab - An elementary school.

mangal - Water-heating equipment made of copper.

Matrakchi Nasuh - A Bosnian-born, highly educated man (1480-1564), who worked in the Ottoman state organization. He had significant geographic, mathematical, mapping and military knowledge. He is also a significant miniature painter who is known for his plasticity and map-like miniatures.

mihrab - A prayer niche in the wall of a mosque indicating the direction of mecca to the congregation.

Mimar Sinan - Chief architect of the Ottoman Empire (1490k-1588), defined the classical style of the Ottoman Era.

minaret - A tower attached to a mosque from which the call to prayer is given.

minber - A 'pulpit' in a mosque usually beside the mihrab.

nahiye - An administrative territory, part of a *sanjak*.

naval stone - See *göbek tashi.*

opeion - A larger size of opening on a cupola which is also covered; skylight.

palisade - A fortification with wooden walls.

pasha - Ottoman honarary title given to provincial governors in the occupied territories.

pendetive - A triangular element taken from a sphere, used when a square ground plan must be covered with a dome. In the corners beneath the dome, the pendetive bridges the angular and curved elements.

qadi - An Ottoman judge with a central role in civil law.

Qusair Amra - An 8th-century Umayyad desert castle in the territory of today's Jordan. The castle contains a bath, in which frescoes also depict humans.

Safavid - Persian dynasty from 1501-1722.

sanjak - Ottoman administrative unit, part of a province.

saray - Palace.

Seljuk - Turkish dynasty. An empire that enjoyed its heyday in the 11th century and stretched from Anatolia in Persia to Central Asia.

skylights - Openings in the ceilings of Turkish baths, they come in many shapes and sizes including: octagonal, circular square or hexagonal.

Sokollu family - One of the 16th century's most important Ottoman families, they came originally from Bosnia with several members finding their way into the service of the Sultan as child tax. Amongst them were several grand viziers. Family members included a Beylerbey of Buda, Mustafa, (1566-78), Ferhad (1588-90), Mehmedpashazade Vezier Hasan Pasha (1593-94), Lala Mehmed Pasha (1599-1600, 1601-1602).

stalactite - A dangling limestone deposit. Similarly, in Ottoman architecture, a common architectural ornament.

tekke - Monastery.

trough vault- A vaulted ceiling made from brick, somewhere in style between a barrel vault and a cloister vault.

türbe - a grave, a memorial building, mausoleum.

vakf - A charity created with a specific goal in mind (eg. the running of a mosque). In the interests of funding the given project, economic activities were attached to it, e.g. baths, land, tax on villages.

vilayet - Province.

Index of Illustrations

Figures 12–13.

The Blue Mosque (Sultan Ahmed Mosque) in Istanbul and an interior view, 1609-1616. Photo by Adrienn Papp.

Figure 14.

Inner courtyard of a madrasa (school). Kurshumliya Madrasa, Sarajevo, 1537. Photo by Gyöngyi Kovács.

Figure 15.

Depiction of a caravanserai (inn) from the travel journal of Salomon Schweigger, 1639, p. 40. Source: https://archive.org/details/einnewereissbes00schwgoog

Figure 16.

Dervish monastery (*tekke*) in Blagaj, Bosnia, late 15th – early 16th century. Photo by Gyöngyi Kovács

Figure 17.

The mausoleum of Sultan Süleyman in Istanbul, 1550–1557. Photo by Adrienn Papp.

Figure 18.

Representation of the Beylerbey's Palace in Timișoara in a drawing by Ferenc Wathay, 1604–1606 (section). Hungarian Academy of Sciences Library and Archive M Cod 4r 29.

Figure 19.

The Süleymaniye complex of buildings (exterior) floorplan, 1550–1557. 1. Mosque. 2. The mausoleum of Süleyman. 3. The mausoleum of Hürrem. 4. Koran recitation school. 5. Public fountain. 6–9., 15–16., 18–19. Schools, various types of madrasa. 9. The remains of a medical school. 10. Infirmary. 11. Poorhouse. 12. Guesthouse. 13. The tomb of Mimar Sinan. 14. Janissary Agha's residence. 17. Baths. Source: https://archnet.org/sites/2024/publications/1446

Figure 20.

The Rumelian Castle on the banks of the Bosporus in Istanbul, 15th century. Photo by Adrienn Papp.

Figure 21.

The 16th-century Old Bridge in Mostar, Bosnia. Tivadar Csontváry Kosztka: Roman bridge at Mostar, 1903. Janus Pannonius Museum. Source: https://upload.wikimedia.org/wikipedia/commons/1/18/Roman_Bridge_at_Mostar_1903.jpg

Figure 22.

Engraving of the Buda gunpowder mill by Ludwig Rohbock, mid-19th century. Source: Hunfalvy 1859.

Figure 23.

The Yakovali Hasan Pasha Mosque. Pécs, early 17th century. Photo by Róbert Hack.

Figure 24.

Interior of the Yakovali Hasan Pasha Mosque. Photo: Róbert Hack

Figure 25.

The restored *mihrab* at the Uzicheli Hadji Ibrahim Mosque (early 17th century). Photo by Adrienn Papp.

Figure 26.

The mausoleum of Gül Baba in Buda, 1543-1548. Photo by Adrienn Papp.

Figure 39.

Bathing woman in an 18th-century depiction. Miniature painting by Husein Fazil bin Tahir Enderuni. In: Huban-name ve Zenanname, 1793. İstanbul Üniversitesi Kütüphanesi/British Library. Source: http://home.earthlink.net/~alqurtubiyya/18/kultur-18.html

Figure 40.

Turkish baths in Ottoman Hungary. Map by Béla Nagy.

Figure 41.

Turkish baths in Buda. Map by Béla Nagy.

Figure 42.

Excavation of the Turkish baths in Pécs. Plan by Béla Nagy.

Figure 43.

Excavation of the Turkish baths in Eger. Plan by Béla Nagy

Figure 44.

Excavation of the Turkish baths in Esztergom. Plan by Béla Nagy.

Figure 45.

Excavation of the Turkish baths in Pest. Plan by Béla Nagy.

Figure 46.

Excavation of the Turkish baths in Székesfehérvár. Plan by Béla Nagy.

Figure 47.

The distribution of Ottoman buildings in Buda. 1. Castle hill. 2. Large suburb. 3. The suburb of Debbaghane. 4. The area of Alhéviz in the Middle Ages. 5. Baruthane. 6. The Beylerbey's Palace. 7. Bridge. 8. Bath. 9. Monastery (*tekke*). 10. Newly built mosque. 11. Mosque adapted from a Christian church. 12. Madrasa. 13. mausoleum. 14. Caravanserai (inn). 15. Warehouse. Plan by Adrienn Papp

Figure 48.

Pécs on Joseph de Haüy's map, 1687. 1. The Kasim Pasha Mosque. 2. The Kasim Pasha Baths. 3. The Ferhad Pasha Mosque. 4. The Ferhad Pasha Baths. 5. The Memi Pasha Mosque. 6. The Memi Pasha Baths. National Széchényi Library, Archive of Maps, inv. no. TM 894.

Figure 49.

View of Eger, 1687. The red arrow points to the location of the steam baths. An unknown German master, Wahre Fürstellung... Vestlung Erla, im Jahr Christi 1687. den 17 Decembris. The Historical Portrait Gallery of the Hungarian National Museum, inv. no. T.231.

Figure 50.

The ruins of the Ottoman era baths in Székesfehérvár. Photo by Róbert Kassay.

Figure 51.

The ruins of the Valide Sultan Baths in Eger. Archive photo. The István Dobó Castle Museum Eger, inv. no. RA510.

Figure 66.
Stalactite decoration in the hot room at the Császár Baths. Photo by Adrienn Papp.
Figure 67.
Stepped decoration around the doorway to the hot room at the Császár Baths. Photo by Adrienn Papp.
Figure 68.
Survey drawings of the vaulting at the Császár Baths, 1974. Drawing by Zsuzsanna Kuczogi. Budapest History Museum, Department of the Mediaeval Era, Archive of Drawings, inv. no. 11864.
Figure 69.
Restored window bars excavated from beside the Rác Baths. Photo by Bence Tihanyi.
Figure 70.
Schematic drawings of the baths of Buda from the Luigi Ferdinando Marsigli collection, late 17th century. Source: Veress 1906, p. 139.
Figure 71.
One of the *iwans* at the restored Császár Baths. Photo: Adrienn Papp
Figure 72.
Portrait of Mimar Sinan, 16th century. Source: https://hu.wikipedia.org/wiki/Szin%C3%A1n#/media/File:Arolsen_Klebeband_02_327.jpg
Figure 73.
Drawing of the Császár Baths by Fischer von Erlach, early 18th century. Budapest History Museum, Engravings Archive, inv. no. 10.960.
Figure 74.
Plan of the sawmill built beside the Rudas Baths in the 18th century, 1712. Budapest City Archive, inv. no. XV.302. BMT140.
Figure 75.
The 19th-century plan for rebuilding the Rudas Baths. Budapest City Archive, inv. no. XV.17.d.328.167.
Figure 76.
The Rudas Baths in Buda. Photo by Gyöngyi Kovács.
Figure 77.
Panoramic view of the eight columns in the hot room of the restored Rudas Baths. Photo: Budapest Spas cPLC.
Figure 78.
Floorplan of the Rudas Baths. 1-2. Warm areas. 3. Hot area. 4. Toilet. Survey drawing by Zsolt Viemann and Adrienn Papp.
Figure 79.
The Rudas Baths following damage inflicted during the Second World War. Kiscelli Museum of the Budapest History Museum, inv. no. 26.698.

Figure 93.

Aerial view of the Rác Baths as they are today. The dome behind the main entrance shows where the Turkish baths stood within the modern building complex. Photo: Civertan.

Figure 94.

The hot room of the Rác Baths following restoration. Source: https://hu.wikipedia.org/wiki/R%C3%A1c_gy%C3%B3gyf%C3%BCrd%C5%91#/media/File:R%C3%A1c_Gy%C3%B3gyf%C3%BCrd%C5%91,_Budapest_02.jpg

Figure 95.

The floorplan of the Rác Baths. 1. Entrance Hall. 2. Warm room. 2b: Pool in the warm room. 3. Toilet. 4. Hot room. 5. Private bath (the coloured arrow indicates the entrance). Plan by Zsolt Viemann and Adrienn Papp.

Figure 96.

The reconstruction of the Rác Baths. Created by Balázs Szőke and Balázs Szakonyi (Pazirik Ltd.)

Figure 97.

The warm room at the Rác Baths: Ottoman era niche and pool. Photo by Adrienn Papp.

Figure 98.

The Rác Baths rebuilding plan from 1890, in which the demolition of the dome to the private bath is represented. Hubert and Móry. Budapest City Arcive, plans registered to plot 5973.

Figure 99.

The Király Baths, Buda. Source: www.kiralyfurdo.hu

Figure 100.

The Király Baths survey plan from 1955. Budapest History Museum, Department of the Mediaeval Era, Archive of Drawings, inv. no. 3901.

Figure 101.

Research on the Király Baths in 1954–1959. Budapest City Archive, inv. no. XV.17.e.306.

Figure 102.

The Király Baths in the 1960s, following refurbishment. The Hungarian Museum of Architecture and Heritage Protection Documentation Centre Photographic Archive, inv. no. 69126.

Figure 103.

Ottoman era window uncovered during restoration work at the Király Baths. Budapest History Museum, Department of the Mediaeval Era, Photographic Archive, inv. no. 17.406.

Figure 104.

The original flooring and wall fountain of the Ottoman era hot room at the Király Baths. Budapest History Museum, Department of the Mediaeval Era, inv. no. 17.415.

Figure 105.

The hot room at the Király Baths as it is today. Photo: Budapest Spas cPLC.

Figure 120.
Esztergom, the Franciscan Bastion (1), the tower of the Héviz baths (2), and the Héviz fortifications (3). 'A' marks the remains of the Mustafa Pasha (?) Baths, 'B' marks the site of the small thermal baths. After István Horváth. MRT 5, p. 115, figure 17.

Figure 121.
The line of the excavated interior walls of the Esztergom thermal baths (17th century). Photo by István Horváth.

Figure 122.
Exterior of the excavated 17th-century thermal baths in Esztergom. Photo by István Horváth.

Figure 123.
Pest, the double baths as they appeared during the excavation. Photo by Bence Tihanyi.

Figure 124.
Pest, the floorplan of the double baths. 1. Entrance hall. 2. Warm room. 3. Hot room. 4. Cistern. 5. Heating area. 6. The remainder of the ruins of the baths. By Zsolt Viemann.

Figure 125.
Pest, Ottoman era remains of marble floor in the hot area of the double baths. Photo by Bence Tihanyi.

Figure 126.
Buda, 1973 survey drawing of the ruins of the Toygun Pasha Baths. 1. Ottoman era walls. 2. Foundations of the floor heating. 3. Clay filling. Budapest History Museum, Department of the Mediaeval Era, Archive of Drawings, inv. no. 11643.

Figure 127.
The Toygun Pasha Baths, probably the foundations of the hot room. Budapest History Museum Data Archive, inv. no. 43-75.

Figure 128.
Survey drawing made during the excavation of the Toygun Pasha Baths. Budapest History Museum, Department of the Mediaeval Era, Archive of Drawings, inv. no. 11644.

Figure 129.
Pécs, survey of the Ferhad Pasha Baths from 1885. Source: Szőnyi 1928, p. 37. https://adtplus.arcanum.hu/hu/view/Historia_01_1928/

Figure 130.
Babócsa, the steam baths during excavation (1988). Photo by Kálmán Magyar.

Figure 131.
Babócsa, steam baths floorplan. Source: Magyar 1990, figure 32.

Acknowledgements

I have many people to thank for the creation of this volume. First of all, Gyöngyi Kovács, who came up with the idea of reworking my doctoral thesis as part of the Hereditas Series. Without her selfless professional and editorial help my work could not have been published.

I would like to thank Balázs Sudár for our discussions of many historical issues across the decades of our professional relationship, as well as for his professional revision of this volume.

I owe great thanks to the art historian Judit Lászay, my research partner in excavating the baths of Buda, for all our work together!

The excavations in Budapest form the backbone of this subject, to which much other research has been associated. The management of the Budapest Historical Museum has always been supportive in this, and I would like to take this opportunity to express my gratitude to them.

Without the expertise and patience of Archaeolingua Publishers and all of their staff, without all their careful planning, editing and preparation work there would be no book for the Reader now to hold.

I am grateful to the members of my family who have accepted the huge amount of time that my writing this book has taken from them, and also for their help in my work.

To deepen my knowledge of the topic I participated in several foreign study tours, for which I thank the Klebelsberg Grant and the Turkish Cultural Foundation scholarship for their financial support.